Abdominal Imaging

pocket tutor

JP

Abdominal Imaging

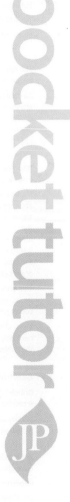

Rakesh Sinha FRCR FICR MD

Consultant Radiologist and Assistant Professor
Warwick Hospital and Medical School
Warwick, UK

JP
medical
publishers

© 2011 JP Medical Ltd.

Published by JP Medical Ltd, 83 Victoria Street, London, SW1H 0HW, UK

Tel: +44 (0)20 3170 8910 Fax: +44 (0)20 3008 6180

Email: info@jpmedpub.com Web: www.jpmedpub.com

ISBN: 978-1-907816-04-8

British Library Cataloguing in Publication Data
A catalogue record for this book is available from the British Library

Library of Congress Cataloging in Publication Data
A catalog record for this book is available from the Library of Congress

JP Medical Ltd is a subsidiary of Jaypee Brothers Medical Publishers (P) Ltd, New Delhi, India (www.jaypeebrothers.com).

Publisher:	Richard Furn
Development Editor:	Paul Mayhew
Copy Editor:	Jane Sugarman
Design:	Pete Wilder, Designers Collective Ltd

Typeset, printed and bound in India.

Preface

With the advent of new imaging modalities the field of abdominal imaging has undergone rapid changes in recent years. However, traditional examinations such as abdominal radiography and barium studies are still used for a variety of conditions. A good working knowledge of common manifestations of disease in both older and new modalities is therefore vital for students and clinicians.

This book starts with a concise overview of abdominal anatomy, then provides a step-by-step guide to interpreting normal imaging results before demonstrating the appearance of key abnormalities. The book then presents concise, practical information on common abdominal conditions that may be encountered in routine medical or surgical practice, each one illustrated by radiological images of the highest quality. Key facts and treatment information are provided for each condition, and a list of key imaging features is included. To facilitate visual understanding, these features are labelled on the corresponding images, along with anatomical landmarks and other notable aspects.

It is hoped that the book will serve as a handy companion for quick reference during teaching and ward rounds, and as a revision tool before examinations. Although primarily aimed at medical students and radiology trainees, the book will also be useful to all physicians and surgeons requiring a pocket-sized guide to abdominal imaging.

Rakesh Sinha

Contents

Acknowledgements

I would like to thank my colleagues at the Radiology Department, Warwick Hospital and also colleagues at South Warwickshire Foundation for their encouragement, help and advice.

I would especially like to thank the editorial team at JP Medical, London for their expertise and help during the production of this book.

Finally I would like to thank my wife and family for their help and support during the writing and production of this book.

Dedication

This book is dedicated to Dr Jogendra P Sinha, Emeritus Professor of Radiology, a role model for generations of residents over several decades.

First principles

1.1 Anatomy

For convenience the abdominal cavity is divided into nine segments (**Figure 1.1**). These regions can be demarcated on an abdominal radiograph by drawing a horizontal line through the 9th ribs and the pelvic brim, and two vertical lines from the centre of the costal cartilage of the 9th rib to the middle of the inguinal ligament. The organs (**Figure 1.2**) contained in these segments are as follows:

- **Right hypochondrium**: gallbladder, right lobe of liver, duodenum, hepatic flexure of colon, upper pole of right kidney and pancreatic head
- **Epigastrium**: stomach, pancreatic body, left lobe of liver
- **Left hypochondrium**: spleen, splenic flexure of colon, and upper pole of left kidney
- **Right lumbar region**: ascending colon and right kidney

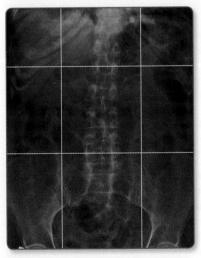

Figure 1.1 The nine abdominal segments. Note normal calcification of the costal cartilages.

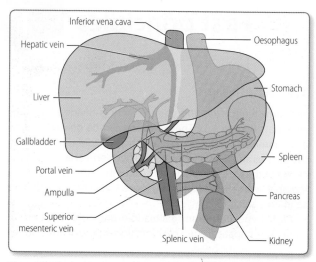

Figure 1.2 The hepatobiliary system, stomach and duodenum. The inferior vena cava (IVC), aorta, superior mesenteric vein and splenic vein join to form the portal vein. The hepatic veins open into the IVC. The common bile duct and pancreatic duct unite to open into the duodenum at the ampulla.

- **Umbilical region:** transverse colon, greater omentum and small bowel
- **Left lumbar region:** descending colon and left kidney
- **Right iliac fossa:** caecum, terminal ileum, appendix and ureter
- **Hypogastrium:** small intestine, bladder and gravid uterus
- **Left iliac fossa:** sigmoid colon, ureter and small bowel.

Abdominal organs

Liver

The liver is the largest organ in the abdomen and consists of a right and a left lobe, divided by the longitudinal fissure, which is seen as a notch in the liver contour (**Figure 1.3**). On radiographs, the liver is seen as a triangular structure on the right; its undersurface may be outlined by fat and is visible across the right hypochondrium or lumbar region. On cross-sectional imaging the liver is seen on the right. If intravenous contrast

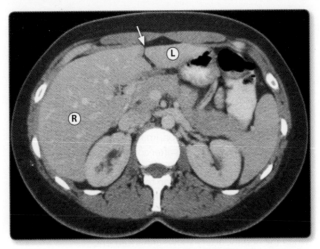

Figure 1.3 CT scan showing the falciform ligament (arrow) dividing the liver into ⓡ the larger right lobe and ⓛ smaller left lobe.

is used, the blood vessels appear of higher signal density than the liver parenchyma.

Lobes of the liver The right lobe is much larger than the left, though this morphology may be reversed in certain pathologies such as cirrhosis, where the right lobe atrophies and appears to be of similar size or smaller than the left lobe. Between 4% and 14% of the population have a prominent inferior extension of the right lower lobe, known as *Riedel's lobe*. This lobe usually extends caudally below the iliac crest.

Two smaller lobes are associated with the right lobe: the quadrate lobe (Latin = square), which is next to the gallbladder bed and the caudate lobe (Latin = tail), which is adjacent to the inferior vena cava (IVC) as it crosses the liver. The normal liver measures up to 13 cm in the midclavicular line (a bilateral vertical line from the middle of the clavicle down the thorax).

Blood supply The liver derives its blood supply from two sources: the hepatic artery and the portal vein.
- The hepatic artery is a branch of the coeliac trunk, which arises from the aorta at the level of the T12 vertebra.

Occasionally the hepatic artery may arise from the superior mesenteric artery.

- The portal vein is formed by the confluence of the splenic vein and the superior mesenteric vein behind the head of pancreas (**Figure 1.4**), and is responsible for 75% of the blood supply to the liver.

This vascular arrangement is physiologically important for radiological imaging. As the portal system is responsible for most of the hepatic blood circulation, imaging of the liver is performed at approximately 60 seconds after contrast injection because this is the amount of time needed for the contrast to pass through the aorta and splanchnic circulation to reach the portal vein (**Figure 1.5**). Primary tumours of the liver are predominantly supplied by the hepatic artery and therefore enhance in the arterial phase, so, to assess the arterial circulation, imaging is done at 30 seconds, when the hepatic artery shows enhancement.

Portal vein velocity and haemodynamics can also be studied on Doppler scans. In the normal state, normal respiratory variation in portal flow is observed, whereas, in diseased states, the variation is often lost and there may be increased/decreased velocity in the portal vein.

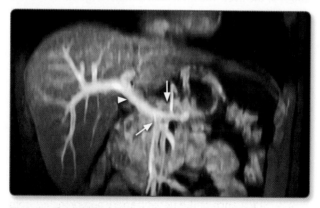

Figure 1.4 Coronal MRI of the liver showing superior mesenteric and splenic veins (arrows) joining to form the portal vein (arrowhead). The portal vein branches are seen within the liver.

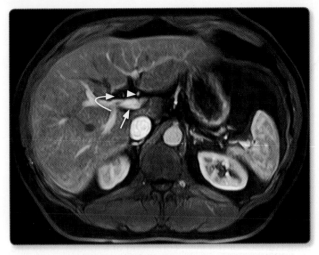

Figure 1.5 Axial MRI at the porta hepatis (hilum of the liver) showing the relationship of the portal vein (arrow) posterior to the hepatic artery (arrowhead) and bile duct (curved arrow).

The venous drainage of the liver is through the hepatic veins into the IVC; these veins can be accessed though the IVC via the jugular or femoral veins for angiography, liver biopsies and hepatic venous pressure measurements.

Pancreas

The pancreas consists of a head, body and tail and is situated transversely across the posterior wall of the abdomen, with its body at the level of T12 (**Figure 1.6**). The head of the pancreas is curved on itself and located along the concavity of the second and third parts of the duodenum. The body of the pancreas is covered anteriorly by layers of the transverse mesocolon and posterior surface of the stomach. Therefore inflammation of the pancreas can involve the colon via the mesocolon and the stomach bed. The pancreas is supplied by the pancreaticoduodenal branch of the hepatic artery and branches from the splenic arteries. Its venous drainage is into the splenic and superior mesenteric veins.

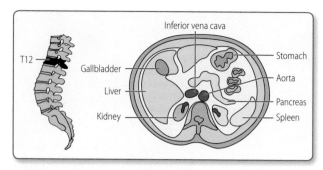

Figure 1.6 Axial section at T12 level showing liver, pancreas, gallbladder, kidneys, aorta and inferior vena cava.

Gallbladder

The gallbladder is a pear-shaped structure located on the undersurface of the liver, consisting of a fundus, body and neck. It is a storage organ for bile produced by the liver, and drains via the cystic duct into the common hepatic duct to form the common bile duct (CBD). The common hepatic duct is formed by the union of the right and left hepatic ducts (**Figure 1.7**). The CBD joins the pancreatic ducts and opens at the duodenal ampulla. It lies to the right of the hepatic artery and in front of the portal vein as it descends to open out at the ampulla.

Spleen

The spleen is an oblong organ located in the left hypochondrium beneath the left 10th rib and hemidiaphragm posterolateral to the gastric fundus (**Figure 1.8**). It is attached to the stomach by the gastrosplenic ligaments, which contain the vascular supply consisting of the splenic artery and veins. The spleen is usually <12 cm in length in an adult, and the splenic vein measures up to 1 cm in diameter. The most inferior surface of the spleen abuts the phrenicocolic ligament, a peritoneal fold that marks the anatomical splenic flexure of the colon.

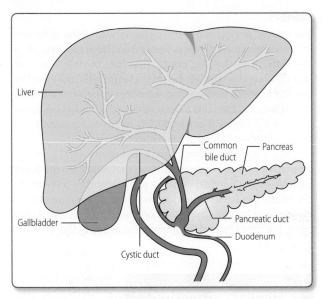

Figure 1.7 The biliary, cystic and pancreatic ducts.

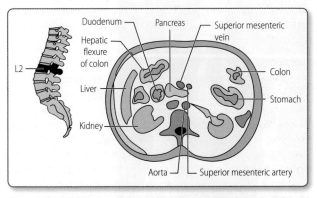

Figure 1.8 Axial section at L2 level showing liver, head of pancreas, kidneys, aorta, inferior vena cava, superior mesenteric vessels and spleen.

Kidneys

The kidneys are located at the posterior wall of the abdomen in the retroperitoneal region. They extend from approximately the 11th rib to the iliac crests. The right kidney is located slightly lower than the left due to the large size of the liver. The external or lateral border is convex, whereas the internal border is concave, and contains a deep notch, which is known at the hilum of the kidney (**Figure 1.9**). The renal vessels, nerves and uterus enter the kidney at the hilum.

The adult kidney varies in length between 8 and 12 cm. The arterial supply is via the renal arteries that arise from the aorta. Each renal artery divides into four or five branches on entering the hilum. The ureters run downwards from the hilum to the bladder and in their course rest on the psoas muscles. At the pelvic brim they cross the common iliac artery before entering the bladder.

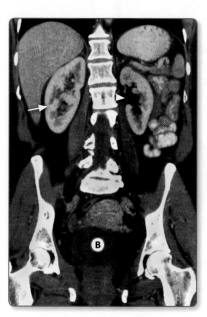

Figure 1.9 Coronal CT image showing the kidneys (arrow) and bladder (**B**). The hilum of the left kidneys is visible (arrowhead).

Stomach and duodenum

The stomach is situated mainly in the left hypochondrium and epigastrium (**Figure 1.10**). It consists of the fundus, body and antrum. The distal-most part of the stomach is the pyloric canal, which communicates with the first part of the duodenum. The lesser curvature of the stomach extends from the oesophageal to the pyloric orifice, along the upper border of the organ, and is attached to the undersurface of the liver via the lesser omentum; the greater curvature is along the outer border and gives attachment to the deep greater omentum. The stomach is supplied by the right gastroepiploic branches of the hepatic and the left gastroepiploic branches of the splenic arteries.

Small intestine

At between 3 and 7 metres, the adult small intestine consists of:
- approximately 26 cm of duodenum (Latin for 12, i.e. its length in fingerwidths),
- 2.5 m of jejunum (Latin: fasting, as it is found empty at death) and
- 2–4 m of ileum (Latin: flank).

The small intestine is coiled centrally, with the shorter colon framing it as it extends clockwise around the abdomen (**Figure 1.11**).

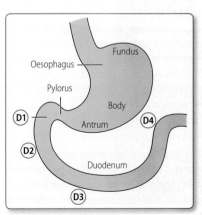

Figure 1.10 The stomach and duodenum, with the four sections of the duodenum labelled D1–D4.

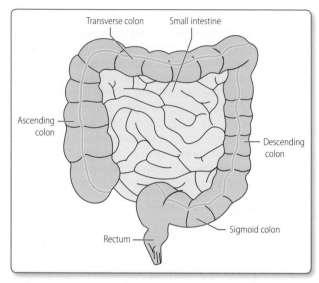

Figure 1.11 The small and large intestine.

Duodenum The duodenum is the shortest and widest part of the small intestine, has no mesenteric attachment and is mostly retroperitoneal.

It consists of four parts (D1-D4):
- D1 (the duodenal cap) communicates with the pylorus
- D2 is vertical and retroperitoneal, passing downward in front of the right kidney to the level of L3. It is into this second section that the common and pancreatic ducts empty
- D3 is horizontal in orientation and crosses the front of the spine, in front of the aorta and IVC
- D4 emerges from the retroperitoneum and joins the jejunum at the level of L1-2.

Jejunum and ileum The jejunum is generally wider than the ileum and contains numerous mucosal folds. The narrower ileum also has many folds and villi for its absorption function, and occupies the hypogastric and right iliac regions. In terms of vasculature, branches of the coeliac artery supply the stomach and duodenum, whereas the superior mesenteric artery supplies the rest of the small intestine, as well as the colon up to the splenic flexure.

Colon

The colon starts at the caecum, where it communicates with the terminal ileum via the ileocaecal valve, and extends clockwise 1.5 m around the abdomen to the rectum. The colon is larger in diameter and more fixed in position than the small intestine, and has characteristic small pouches, called 'haustra', caused by sacculations (folding) of the colonic wall. The caecum is located in the right iliac fossa (**Figure 1.12**). The ileocaecal valve is usually on the posteromedial wall of the caecum, and the appendix approximately 2 cm below the valve.

The ascending colon is located along the right flank and continues as the transverse colon, which crosses the abdomen and then descends along the left lumbar region to the left iliac

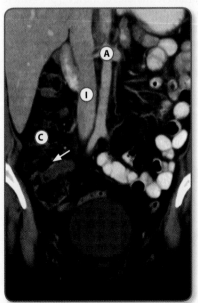

Figure 1.12 Coronal CT image showing the ascending colon Ⓒ and the ileocaecal junction (arrow). The aorta Ⓐ and inferior vena cava Ⓘ are seen in the midline along with small bowel loops in the left side Ⓛ of the abdomen.

fossa. The ascending and descending portions of the colon are retroperitoneal and therefore fixed in position. Conversely, the transverse colon, caecum and sigmoid colon are attached to their respective mesocolon (a double layer of peritoneum) and hang freely within the abdominal cavity. Therefore, these segments may be tortuous or mobile. At the left iliac fossa the colon becomes more tortuous as it forms the sigmoid colon. It enters the pelvis and descends along the posterior wall and presacral space, to form the rectum and anal canal.

The blood supply of the colon distal to the splenic flexure is via the inferior mesenteric artery. The rectum also gets blood supply from the superior and inferior rectal arteries of the iliac blood vessels.

Abdominal vasculature

The abdominal aorta starts at the diaphragmatic opening at the level of the T12 vertebral. It usually descends slightly to the left of the vertebral column and terminates at the level of L4 where it divides into the two common iliac arteries (**Figure 1.13**). The major visceral branches of the aorta are the coeliac axis, superior and inferior mesenteric arteries, suprarenal arteries, renal arteries and spermatic arteries. Parietal branches (parietal = relating to the walls of a part or cavity) are the phrenic, lumbar and sacral arteries.

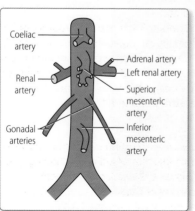

Figure 1.13 The abdominal aorta with branches.

Coeliac artery

Renal artery

Gonadal arteries

Adrenal artery

Left renal artery

Superior mesenteric artery

Inferior mesenteric artery

1.2 Imaging modalities

Radiographs

Radiographs are formed by X-rays passing through the body and forming a latent image on the film or sensor placed behind. Different tissues of the body absorb different amounts of X-ray photons, producing different densities on the image – a 'shadow' of tissues. Bones absorb most of the X-ray photons because they have a higher electron density than soft tissues. When the film is developed, the parts of the image corresponding to higher X-ray exposure are dark, leaving a white shadow of bones on the film.

X-rays are widely used in medicine for producing images of the body and also for certain treatments (radiotherapy). Their beneficial use must always be weighed against the potential harm they cause as a form of ionising radiation, which can lead to cellular destruction and mutations in DNA. The biological effect of radiation on human tissue is measured as the equivalent dose and expressed in sieverts (symbol: Sv). In general, routine radiographs do not impart significant radiation dose; however, CT, nuclear and interventional examinations impart significant radiation to patients, so these high radiation dose examinations are performed only after due justification and their perceived benefit over risk to the patient (**Table 1.1**).

> **Background**
>
> X-rays were discovered in 1895 by Professor Wilhelm Conrad Röntgen, who won the first Nobel Prize in physics for his discovery. Röntgen noticed a glow emitted by a cathode-ray tube, which caused a fluorescent plate to glow. These invisible emissions that could penetrate solid objects were termed 'X-rays'. He used the rays to make images of coins inside a wooden box, and then of the human body. He allowed radiographs of his wife's hand to be published in newspapers, creating a worldwide demand for X-rays.

Use of contrast agents

Several other techniques are used to enhance the normal X-ray examination. For example, injection of iodine-containing intravenous contrast can delineate the vasculature (iodine, being dense, outlines the blood vessels against the soft tissues). This technique is known as angiography (**Figure 1.14**).

Region imaged/ diagnostic procedure	Dose (mSv)	Time to receive same dose from background radiation	Risk of fatal cancer
Barium enema	7	3.2 years	1:3000
Barium meal	3	16 months	1:6700
IVU	2.5	14 months	1:8000
Barium swallow	1.5	8 months	1:13,000
Lumbar spine	1.3	7 months	1:15,000
Abdomen	0.7	4 months	1:30,000
Pelvis	0.7	4 months	1:30,000
Thoracic spine	0.7	4 months	1:30,000
Hip	0.3	7 weeks	1:67,000
Cervical spine	0.08	2 weeks	1:200,000
Chest (single posterroanterior film)	0.02	3 days	1 in a million
Teeth (single bitewing)	<0.01	<1.5 days	1 in a few million
Limbs and joints	<0.01	<1.5 days	1 in a few million
CT of abdomen or pelvis	10	4.5 years	1:2000

Table 1.1 Typical radiation doses during diagnostic radiography.

Injection of contrast and acquisition of images after a delay of 5–30 min allow delineation of the urinary system as the kidneys excrete the iodinated contrast. This examination is termed 'intravenous urography' (IVU) (**Figure 1.15**).

The gastrointestinal (GI) tract can be delineated by using barium sulphate solution. Barium, as a dense, inert, metallic ion, outlines the GI tract on radiographs. These procedures are called barium swallow (oesophagus), barium follow-through (small intestine) and barium enema (colon) examinations (**Figure 1.16**).

Fluoroscopy

Fluoroscopy is another technique in which X-rays are used to image the body in real time. In this type of examination,

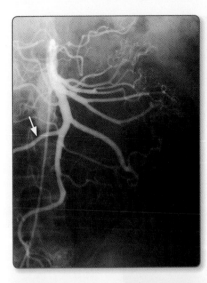

Figure 1.14 Angiogram of the superior mesenteric artery after injection of dye through a transfermoral catheter shows its jejunal and ileal branches. The ileocolic branch is marked (arrow).

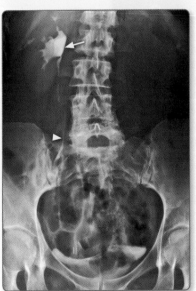

Figure 1.15 IVU image taken at 10 minutes demonstrating the renal calyces (arrow) and ureter (arrowhead) outlined by iodinated contrast. Note the patient has only a single kidney.

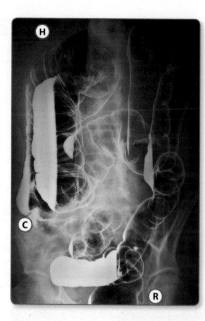

Figure 1.16 Abdominal radiograph after a barium enema (instillation of barium per rectum) showing the colon in its entirety. (H) hepatic flexure, (C) caecum, (R) rectum.

continuous X-ray exposure of the body (e.g. 2 frames/s or more) produces a cine image. For example, fluoroscopy may be used in assessing peristalsis of the bowel on a barium follow-through examination or the swallowing mechanism in a barium swallow examination. Fluoroscopy is also particularly useful in guiding interventional procedures such as biopsies and drainages.

Computed tomography

Intravenous and oral contrast are usually administered during abdominal CT examinations to delineate the GI tract and vasculature. Intravenous contrast is particularly useful in assessing the vascularity or enhancement patterns of tumours and abnormal tissue. Intravenous contrast contains iodine, which appears hyperdense on CT images so blood vessels appear dense. Recent advances in CT technology allow scans to be acquired within seconds and powerful software allows detailed three-dimensional images of the body.

The main clinical indications for CT is in the setting of acute abdominal presentations (e.g. trauma, bowel obstruction, renal colic), cancer staging and diagnosis, follow-up imaging of cancer after treatment to assess response and during guidance for biopsy or drainages.

Ultrasound

Ultrasound (US) uses high-frequency sound waves (>2 mHz) to visualise body tissues with real-time sonographic images. It was originally developed from

Background

The British scientist Sir Godfrey Hounsfield invented the first prototype of the CT scanner in the 1970s after having the idea of trying to determine what was in a lunch box by taking X-ray slices from all possible angles. Similarly, CT images are produced by acquiring slices of X-ray images in 360° and reconstructing them to form the complete image **(Figure 1.17)**.

The first clinical image of a patient with a suspected brain lesion was acquired in 1972 under the guidance of the radiologist Dr James Ambrose, working with Sir Hounsfield (he recalled that both he and Hounsfield felt like footballers who had just scored the winning goal!). As his legacy, the density of tissue on CT images is measured in Hounsfield units (HU), with water having a value of 0 HU. Fat and air have negative Hounsfield values, whereas dense objects have positive Hounsfield values.

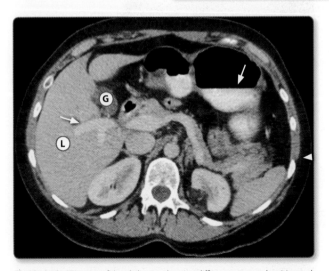

Figure 1.17 CT image of the abdomen showing different contrast densities and accurate anatomical delineation of abdominal organs. L = Liver; G= Gallbladder. Iodinated contrast in the portal vein and in stomach (arrows).

military SONAR technology used in the navy, and is now one of the most widely used diagnostic tools. A handheld transducer (probe) emits high frequency sound waves (above 20 kHz) that are reflected to varying degrees by the body tissues. These reflected echoes are sensed by the same probe and used to create the image. Dense tissues and material reflect more soundwaves (hy-

Guiding principle

A Swiss physicist called Daniel Colladon used a bell under water to decipher the speed of sound in water in the 1820s. His experiments defined the basic physics of sound wave transmission, reception and refraction. The Curie brothers discovered the piezo-electric effect in 1880 and a piezo-electric crystal forms the basic component of ultrasound probes. These crystals produce and receive sound waves and enable measurements of acoustic energy, depth and velocity

perechoic) and hence appear light **(Figure 1.18)**. Conversely, fluid and air reflect less (hypoechoic) and transmit more of the soundwaves and appear dark. The advantages of US include its lack of radiation and the ability to visualise tissue in real time.

Doppler imaging

US examinations can be supplemented with Doppler scans that assess blood flow in body tissues **(Figure 1.19)**. Doppler

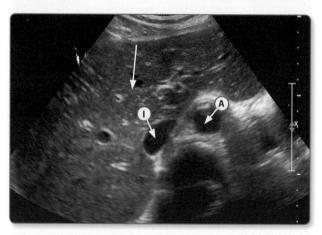

Figure 1.18 US image of the right upper quadrant showing the moderate reflectivity of the liver (arrow). (**I**) inferior vena cava, (**A**) aorta are labelled.

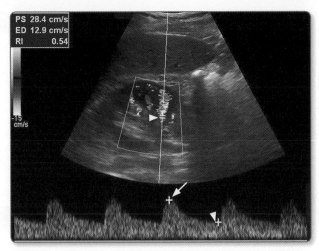

Figure 1.19 Doppler scan of the renal artery showing normal flow. The cursor for Doppler measurement has been placed on the renal artery (arrowhead). Trace shows peak systolic flow (long arrow) and end diastolic flow (short arrow) values.

imaging uses the physical principle of the Doppler effect to assess whether blood is moving towards or away from the probe, and its relative velocity. By convention, blood flowing towards the probe is labelled red whereas blood flowing away from it is labelled blue on US images.

Magnetic resonance imaging

First used in 1977, magnetic resonance imaging (MRI) uses the spin properties of hydrogen nuclei to generate images. It uses a powerful magnetic field to align all the hydrogen atoms in the body. Once aligned the atoms have a net longitudinal magnetic moment. A switching radiofrequency pulse is then used to disrupt this alignment. The radiofrequency pulse imparts extra energy to the atoms and they spin out of the longitudinal arrangement into a transverse orientation. Once the pulse is switched off, the hydrogen atoms again realign longitudinally to the magnetic field. In returning from a transverse to a longitudinal orientation, a rotating, diminishing magnetic field is created. The return of the excited nuclei from the high-energy to the low-energy state is associated with the loss of energy to the surrounding nuclei and MR images are based on the observation of this relaxation that takes place after the radio-frequency pulse has stopped.

MR images can be constructed because the protons in different tissues return to their equilibrium state at different rates. By varying imaging parameters such as TR (pulse repetition time) and TE (echo time), it is possible to produce T1- or T2-weighted images. T1 is the spin-lattice or longitudinal relaxation time, and T2 is the spin-spin or transverse relaxation time. Different tissues appear differently in both images:

- fat appears bright on T1-weighted images
- fluid appears bright on T2-weighted images (**Figure 1.20**).

MR scans usually take longer to acquire than CT scans, and assessing one

Clinical insight

A simple reminder for telling the difference between T1 and T2 weighting is "tea for two", i.e. liquids are bright on T2-weighted images.

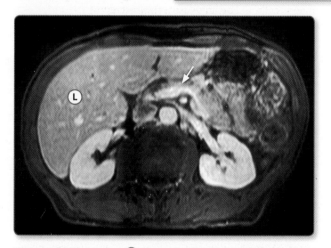

Figure 1.20 MRI of the liver Ⓛ showing enhancement of the portal veins (arrow) and parenchyma. Note the bones are dark (hypointense) as they do not have many unpaired hydrogen ions to produce a signal on images.

organ (such as liver) may take 25–30 min, although MRI provides much greater contrast between the different soft tissues of the body. MR images take longer to acquire because a number of different sequences are required to define anatomical detail, organ-specific sequences and sequences for highlighting specific disease processes. Each individual sequence may take about 5 min and a typical examination may use several sequences. The dynamic enhancement patterns of abdominal organs can also be assessed by using ultrafast sequences. MRI has the advantage over CT and radiographs that ionising radiation is not involved.

MRI with and without contrast agents

Intravenous contrast agents used in MRI contain gadolinium or manganese, which have paramagnetic properties. Unlike CT or US, which use only X-rays or sound waves to generate images, MRI exploits a long list of tissue properties to generate images and thus can be more tissue specific. For example, blood flow within the arteries can be used to generate angiographic images without having to use a contrast agent.

Nuclear imaging

Nuclear imaging relies on specific radionuclides that are injected into the body for production of images. A radionuclide is an atom with an unstable nucleus, which undergoes radioactive decay and in doing so produces ionising radiation such as gamma rays and subatomic particles. These emissions are detected by cameras to produce images. Radionuclides may occur naturally, but can also be artificially produced. Some commonly used radionuclides are isotopes of technetium (^{99m}Tc) and iodine (^{123}I and ^{131}I), thallium-201, gallium-67 and indium-111.

Nuclear imaging shows the physiological function of the system being investigated as opposed to traditional anatomical imaging such as CT or MRI. Nuclear medicine imaging studies are generally more tissue specific, e.g. ^{99m}Tc may be used to visualise bony metastases because it is taken up by metabolically active bone lesions and appears as hot spots on images.

Positron emission tomography–CT (PET-CT) combines PET and CT to acquire images on a single superimposed image. PET is a nuclear imaging technique that produces a three-dimensional image; it uses the radioactive tracer (radionuclide) fluorodeoxyglucose (FDG) as contrast. FDG is taken up by tissues with a high metabolic rate and appears as hot spots on images (**Figure 1.21**). PET-CT has a very high sensitivity in the detection of metastases and tumours (the cells of which are often highly metabolic) compared with other modalities.

Interventional radiology

Abdominal interventions such as biopsies or drainages may be carried out by radiologists under imaging guidance using fluoroscopy, US, CT or MRI. These imaging modalities are typically used to guide needles or catheters into correct anatomical locations. For example US or fluoroscopy may be used to guide puncture of the bile duct in a percutaneous transhepatic

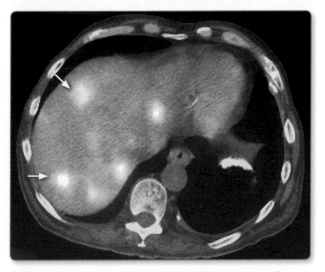

Figure 1.21 PET-CT image of the liver showing multiple metastases as "hot spots" (arrows).

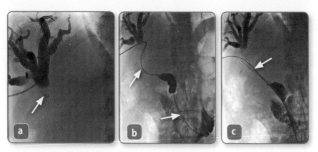

Figure 1.22 (a) Percutaneous cholangiogram (PTC) showing obstruction of bile ducts at hilum (arrow). (b) A guidewire (arrows) has been manipulated through the stricture into the duodenum. (c) A metallic stent (arrow) is being deployed across the stricture.

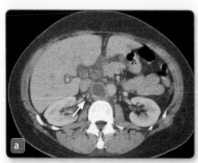

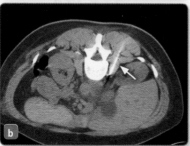

Figure 1.23 (a) CT image showing a small abscess (arrow) between the aorta and inferior vena cava. (b) Needle is seen (arrow) being introduced into the abscess for drainage under CT guidance.

cholangiogram examination (**Figures 1.22** and **1.23**). Imaging is also required for more complex interventions such as placing of stents or angioplasties.

chapter 2

Understanding normal results

2.1 Abdominal radiographs

Introduction

As the X-ray beam passes through the body, it is attenuated to differing degrees by the various body tissues so it produces different densities or shadows on the resultant radiographic image.

- Dense objects appear white as they absorb more of the X-rays, preventing them from reaching the film/detector behind them
- Soft tissues are grey; fat is dark grey
- Air (for example, within the bowel) is black as it only minimally effects attenuation.

It is useful to know the varying degrees that different tissues attenuate X-rays in order to interpret radiographs adequately (**Figure 2.1**). For example, intra-abdominal fat encases most abdominal organs and therefore recognition of typical fat densities against the densities of the organs can help in assessing organ size and morphology.

Abdominal radiographs are routinely performed as an initial investigation in patients with acute abdominal symptoms – an acute intra-abdominal condition of abrupt onset. Such cases of 'acute abdomen' are usually associated with pain due to inflammation, perforation, obstruction, infarction or rupture of abdominal organs. In many abdominal conditions evaluation of the gas pattern, abdominal calcification and mass effects can help diagnose the underlying condition. Furthermore, findings on the abdominal radiograph may guide subsequent imaging, e.g. bowel dilatation may prompt a CT examination to look for the level and cause of bowel obstruction.

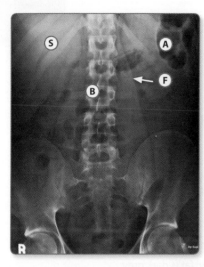

Figure 2.1 Radiograph showing different kinds of densities: (B) bone, (S) soft tissue, (F) fat, (A) air.

Currently abdominal radiographs are of value in patients with acute abdomen, renal colic and suspected bowel obstruction. Their use in other abdominal conditions is of limited value.

Guiding principle

Gas or air produces dark black shadows on radiographs. Bones and metallic objects produce a dense white shadow. Solid organs appear grey whereas fat produces a darker shade of grey in between the density of solid organs and gas.

Fat lines or stripes

There is a considerable amount of fat and adipose tissue between the transverse fascia covering the inner surface of abdominal muscles (rectus abdominis, external and internal oblique muscles) and the peritoneum. On radiographs these appear as linear dark-grey lines and are termed the 'properitoneal fat lines'. They are best seen when tangential to the X-ray beam and therefore best visualised in both flanks (**Figures 2.2** and **2.3**). This is because they

Guiding principle

- Different body tissues cause varying levels of attenuation of the X-ray beam, leading to the perception of different densities on the resultant image
- These differences in density help to identify normal anatomical structures

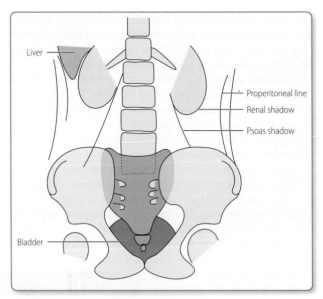

Figure 2.2 Fat lines: Location of properitoneal lines, renal shadow, psoas shadows.

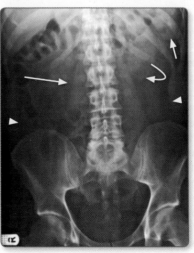

Figure 2.3 Fat lines on abdominal radiograph. Psoas shadow (long arrow), Inferior edge of spleen (short arrow), lower pole of kidney (curved arrow), properitoneal lines (arrowheads).

are seen in relief adjacent to the abdominal muscles (external and internal obliques), which are of soft-tissue density (grey).

It is important to visualise these fat lines because they may be absent or blurred in intra-abdominal diseases:

- **Liver and spleen:** the inferior edge can be seen outlined by mesenteric fat and peritoneal fat stripes. The lower edge of the liver is located approximately 1 cm below the lowest costal margin in the erect posture
- **Kidneys:** these are seen outlined by a darker rim of surrounding retroperitoneal fat
- **Psoas muscles:** on either side of the lumbar spine, the lateral margins of these muscles can be seen in most adults. The psoas muscles diverge from the lower thoracic spine and fan out to the iliac bones. The right psoas outline may be blurred in up to 19% of adults and is seen in only half of children
- **Aorta:** generally not seen separately from the psoas shadow unless it is aneurysmal and contains calcification secondary to atherosclerosis
- **Bladder:** if distended, it can be seen in the pelvis, outlined by intrapelvic fatty tissue

Gas shadows

Normally, gas is present within the stomach and large bowel, whereas only a small amount is seen in the small bowel (**Figures 2.4** and **2.5**).

Faecal matter is often seen intermixed with gas within the colon and, as air and fluid are present in the bowel, fluid levels may also be seen. Fluid levels are classically seen on erect radiographs and formed by the presence of gas and fluid within the bowel lumen. In the erect posture, fluid gravitates to the dependent portion of the bowel, whereas gas collects superiorly and forms a linear opacity at the interface with gas shadows above and soft-tissue density below. Three to five fluid levels <2.5 cm in length may be seen in normal individuals. Usually fluid levels are seen at the first part of the duodenum and in the right iliac fossa at the ileocaecal junction.

When outlined by gas, the small bowel can be identified by the presence of mucosal folds called valvulae conniventes

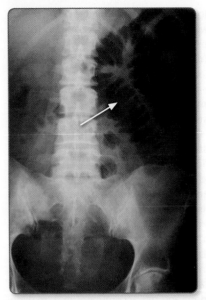

Figure 2.4 Radiograph showing valvulae conniventes in the small bowel (arrow).

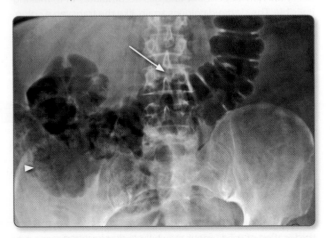

Figure 2.5 Radiograph showing haustrations in the colon (arrow). Faecal matter mixed with air may create mottled densities in the colon as seen in the caecum (arrowhead).

(**Figure 2.4**). These appear as linear or spiral folds crossing the lumen of the bowel; they are closely packed together in the proximal small bowel (jejunum) and more widely spaced in the distal portion (ileum). The normal small bowel should measure <3 cm in diameter. The colon can be identified by its location and the presence of haustrations, which are produced by crescentic indentations of the entire colonic wall; these help to distinguish the large bowel from the small bowel (**Figure 2.5**). It must be remembered that in up to one third of adults the distal descending and sigmoid colon may not contain haustrations.

The ascending and descending colon are retroperitoneal structures and are therefore fairly fixed in position, located along the right and left flanks, respectively. The transverse colon lies across the upper part of the abdomen and, as it hangs on the transverse mesocolon (formed by two layers of peritoneum), it is mobile, located anteriorly in the abdomen. Therefore, in the supine position (method by which most abdominal radiographs are acquired) this segment of the colon becomes non-dependent and gas accumulates in it, making it visible. The sigmoid colon is again, like the transverse colon, attached to its mesentery (sigmoid mesocolon) and may be long and tortuous in some individuals. The colon is variable in size, though a diameter of >5 cm is considered abnormal. The caecum is more distensible, so a diameter of >9 cm is considered abnormal.

Solid organs

Solid organs project as uniform, grey shadows on abdominal radiographs. They are visible because they are outlined by fat.

Abnormal lucencies or calcifications projected over the location of solid organs may help in diagnosing disease, e.g. air shadows (lucent or dark shadows) over the liver may indicate the presence of a liver abscess containing gas, or calcifications (dense or white shadows) over the renal shadow may indicate

> ### Guiding principle
>
> Some institutionalised patients may have large colons measuring up to 10–15 cm in diameter without any obvious clinical symptoms. This is most often due to loss of muscular tone of the bowel caused by neuromuscular degeneration.

the presence of renal stones, which contain calcium and are dense.

With the advent of cross-sectional imaging modalities, abdominal radiographs are generally not used to diagnose pathologies affecting solid organs because internal abnormalities cannot be detected.

Bones and normal calcifications

The lumbar spine, pelvis, hip joints and lower ribs are normally visible on the abdominal radiograph (**Figures 2.6** and **2.7**). Usually calcification may be seen in mesenteric lymph nodes, which typically appear of amorphous density. Calcified venous valves (phleboliths) can also be seen, particularly in the pelvis. They are typically ring shaped with a relatively lucent centre. Calcifications in the costal cartilages are also typically speckled or irregular in appearance.

A step-by-step approach to interpreting abdominal radiographs

Radiographs should be interpreted in a systematic manner, i.e. evaluating the bones, fat lines, soft-tissue shadows and solid

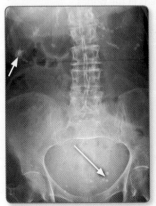

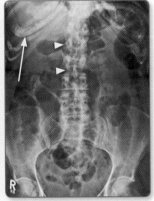

Figure 2.6 Radiograph showing calcification in lymph node (short arrow) and phleboliths (long arrow).

Figure 2.7 Radiograph showing calcifications in the costal cartilage (arrow). Note uniform appearance of the spine with round pedicles (arrowheads).

organs in a consistent order (**Figure 2.8**). One must develop a method of assessing all the information available. A suggested approach is as follows:

> ## Clinical insight
>
> A personal routine should be established while interpreting radiographs. Either one starts by evaluating the bones, fat lines, soft-tissue shadows and solid organs or the other way round. This approach ensures that one does not miss out any abnormalities. With practice, this routine becomes second nature and can be performed quickly.

1. Assess the clinical information at hand. This may help to correlate these findings on the abdominal radiograph
2. Identify fat lines and stripes in both flanks and look for any blurring or obscuration
3. Identify the psoas shadows and fat lines around the kidneys and undersurface of liver and spleen. Assess whether there is enlargement of the liver or spleen or if any of the fat stripes are absent
4. Assess the bowel gas shadows and identify if there is any abnormal dilatation (small bowel >3 cm; large bowel >5 cm)
5. Assess the bones of the spine and pelvis. Identify any abnormally dense or lucent areas in the bones

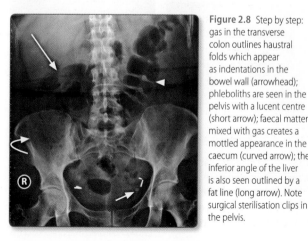

Figure 2.8 Step by step: gas in the transverse colon outlines haustral folds which appear as indentations in the bowel wall (arrowhead); phleboliths are seen in the pelvis with a lucent centre (short arrow); faecal matter mixed with gas creates a mottled appearance in the caecum (curved arrow); the inferior angle of the liver is also seen outlined by a fat line (long arrow). Note surgical sterilisation clips in the pelvis.

6. Next the entire radiograph should be evaluated for any abnormally dense (white) shadows that may represent calcification or stones. If these densities are projected over the kidneys or liver, correlation with clinical information must be sought in order to diagnose renal stones or gallstones

Guiding principle

- An abnormal gas pattern, such as distended bowel loop, can help in the diagnosis of bowel obstruction
- Abnormal calcification over solid organs may indicate presence of stones
- Enlarged organs may indicate an underlying mass lesion

7. Identify any abnormal lucencies (black or dark shadows) over solid organs or in any abnormal locations because these may represent abscesses or extraintestinal air

8. Assess both inguinal regions for any abnormal gas shadows (black) because if present they may represent bowel within an inguinal hernia

9. Identify any surgical clips or sutures (they appear dense or white). This may be useful in cases with suspected bowel obstruction.

Clinical insight

Experience is needed for the interpretation of normal and abnormal gas shadows. The normal appearance of small and large bowel and faecal matter (mottled lucencies) is learnt by spending time visualising the different patterns on normal abdominal radiographs.

The presence of surgical clips in these cases may indicate bowel obstruction secondary to adhesions due to previous surgery. Adhesions are fibrous bands that form between tissues and organs, often as a result of injury during surgery.

2.2 Abdominal ultrasound

Ultrasound is particularly useful for evaluating the hepatobiliary tract, and can detect gallstones with great facility. The gallbladder, bile ducts, pancreas and kidneys can be also readily be examined.

Doppler studies can be performed to assess blood flow velocities in abdominal arteries and veins. Increased blood flow may be seen in cases with inflammation or infections. Narrowing or stenosis of arteries also causes increased velocity of blood flow because, according to Bernoulli's principle, reduction of the cross-sectional area of tubular flow increases the flow velocity. For example, assessment of renal artery flow can be done to check velocity and flow parameters, because renal artery stenosis is an important cause of hypertension.

Liver

Normally the liver has homogeneous echogenicity (echoes are similar throughout the liver) (**Figure 2.9**). This is due to the relatively homogenous nature of liver tissue, consisting of hepatocytes.

The branches of the portal and hepatic veins appear as linear hypoechoic (darker) structures. At the medial edge of the liver is the hilum, which contains the main portal vein, common bile duct and hepatic artery.

The liver normally measures <13 cm in the midclavicular line. The left lobe of the liver is scanned by placing the probe

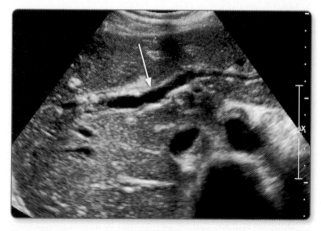

Figure 2.9 US scan showing the liver. Portal vein appears as a hypoechoic tubular structure (arrow).

in the midline in the epigastric region. The right lobe is usually scanned via a right intercostal approach.

Gallbladder

The gallbladder appears as a thin-walled hypoechoic (dark) cyst-like structure and its wall thickness is <3 mm (**Figure 2.10**). It is located below the anteroinferior edge of the liver. Fasting for 4–6 hours is necessary to allow distension of the gallbladder for adequate assessment. The gallbladder is usually scanned via a right intercostal approach or anteriorly via the right lumbar quadrant.

Pancreas

The pancreas is seen in the midline anterior to the aorta and is generally of greater echogenicity compared with the liver (**Figure 2.11**). It is approximately 15 cm long, from head to tail, and is usually seen as a 'J shape', with the loop of the J around the duodenum. Posterior to the pancreas is a tubular hypoechoic structure (splenic vein). The pancreas is scanned by placing the probe in the midline in the epigastric region.

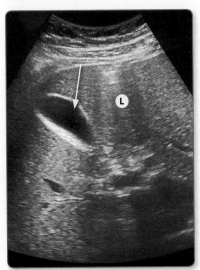

Figure 2.10 US scan showing the gallbladder as a sac-like anechoic structure (arrow) in the right upper quadrant just below the inferior edge of the liver. Ⓛ liver.

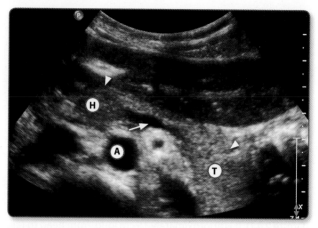

Figure 2.11 US scan showing the pancreas (arrowheads) as a moderately echoic structure anterior to the mesenteric and splenic vein (arrow). (A) aorta, (H) head of pancreas, (T) tail of pancreas.

Kidneys

The kidneys have an inner echogenic (bright) area corresponding to the medulla and an outer relatively echo-poor region corresponding to the cortex (**Figure 2.12**). The medulla contains fat, which causes increased reflectivity of ultrasound waves, leading to an echogenic appearance. Normally the cortex of the kidney is of darker reflectivity than the liver. Increased brightness of the cortex is associated with renal disease. The normal adult kidneys measures between 9 and 11 cm in length. The kidneys are usually scanned by placing the probe on the flanks.

Pelvis

In the pelvis the uterus and ovaries may be assessed by ultrasonography. A full bladder may be necessary to provide an acoustic window to assess pelvic organs (**Figures 2.13** and **2.14**). The pelvic organs are scanned by placing the probe in a suprapubic region and iliac fossae.

Transvaginal scanning is often employed to assess the ovaries and the uterus because using this approach organs can be viewed

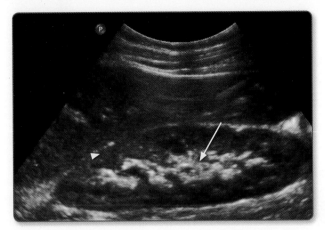

Figure 2.12 US scan of the kidney (arrow) showing hypoechoic cortex (arrowhead) and echogenic medulla (arrow).

closer, in higher resolution. Transrectal ultrasound is performed to assess the prostate and guide prostatic biopsies. Transrectal or endoanal sonography is also performed for assessment of anal sphincter abnormalities. The pelvic organs are scanned by placing the probe in a suprapubic region and iliac fossae.

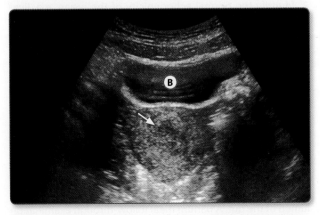

Figure 2.13 US scan showing the uterus (arrow) through the anechoic urinary bladder. **B** bladder.

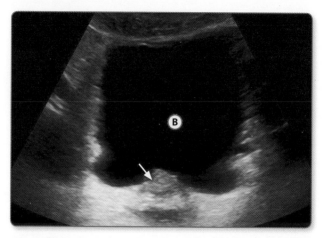

Figure 2.14 US scan showing the prostate gland (arrow) below the base of the bladder (B).

Step-by-step approach to interpreting ultrasound images

1. Identify the organ being examined. On images, labels may be present and position of the probe indicated
2. Identify the normal echogenicity of the organ, e.g. liver and spleen are homogeneous, whereas the kidney has a hypoechoic cortex and echogenic medulla
3. Identify if any low echo areas are present in the solid organs
4. Identify if any echogenic areas are present in the organs associated with shadowing (calculi)
5. Identify if any fluid is present (anechoic areas) surrounding the organs.

2.3 Barium studies

Barium studies are undertaken to evaluate the gastrointestinal (GI) tract using this dense, radio-opaque, inert, metallic ion that, once ingested (as barium sulphate solution), outlines the lumen of the gut. A barium meal follow-through examination is done to visualise the small bowel (**Figure 2.15**), whereas the colon may be evaluated by a barium enema via the rectum (**Figure 2.16**).

CT and MRI have largely replaced barium investigations, although they still play a significant role in the evaluation of paediatric GI tract anomalies and intestinal infections. Barium examinations allow detailed evaluation of mucosal abnormalities, intestinal fold patterns and abnormalities of peristalsis.

The normal small bowel outlined by barium shows the presence of mucosal folds, which are more numerous in the jejunum than in the ileum. Typically the jejunum displays a feathery mucosal pattern whereas the ileum appears more dense and tubular. The ileocaecal junction is situated in the right iliac fossa where contrast passes into the colon. The colon has haustrations rather than mucosal folds, which appear as indentations or undulations in the bowel wall, although the sigmoid may have none. In adults most of the jejunal loops are located in the left upper quadrant

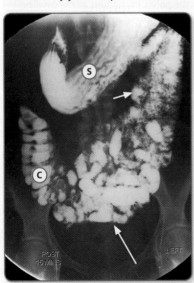

Figure 2.15 Barium meal follow-through examination. Barium outlines the bowel loops: Ⓢ stomach, Ⓒ caecum. Jejunal loops (short arrow) are located in the left upper quadrant and have closely packed mucosal folds, which produce a feathery pattern. Ileal loops are in the pelvis (long arrow) and have less numerous folds.

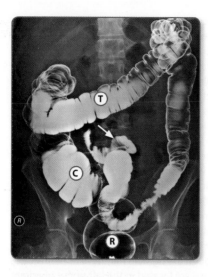

Figure 2.16 Barium enema examination outlines the colon and demonstrates the haustral folds. Ⓒ caecum, Ⓣ transverse colon, Ⓡ rectum. Barium has refluxed into the terminal ileum, which delineates the different mucosal fold pattern of the small bowel (arrow) compared with the colon.

whereas the ileum lies in the pelvis. In children, all the small bowel loops are commonly located in the pelvis.

2.4 CT and MRI

CT scanning is the 'gold standard' imaging modality in the evaluation of the acute abdomen. As X-rays are used to produce CT images, the densities of body tissues follow a similar pattern to that of plain radiographs. Bones appear bright whereas gas appears black. The solid abdominal organs appear of a similar intermediate density. Fat and fluid have densities that are darker than solid organs. CT images are usually obtained in cross-sectional (axial) planes and data can then be reconstructed to produce sagittal or coronal images.

Clinical insight

- Enhancement of body tissue can be measured as a change in the Hounsfield units before and after intravenous contrast administration. Fresh blood (e.g. haemorrhage after trauma) is typically hyperdense, measuring between 100 and 200 HU

- Current generation multidetector CT scanners can obtain images of the entire abdominopelvic region within one breathhold (4-20s), making a rapid overview of the entire abdomen possible even with uncooperative or acutely unwell patients

Densities of body tissues are measured in Hounsfield units (HU); water has the density of 0 HU whereas air has negative density of −500 HU. Dense objects such as bones are >300–400 HU.

Transpyloric plane

At this level (L1 vertebra) on axial images the liver is seen as a triangular structure located in the right sub-

> ### Guiding principle
>
> - MRI and ultrasound do not use X-rays and are therefore non-ionising investigations with no significant adverse effects on patients
> - MRI has high tissue specificity and therefore is highly accurate in detecting pathologies affecting abdominal organs. However, its spatial resolution is less than that of CT and its scanning times are much longer

diaphragmatic space (**Figure 2.17**). The left lobe of the liver extends across the midline to the left. The hepatic vasculature appears denser than the liver due to injection of intravascular contrast. The pancreas is seen in the midline anterior to the portal and coeliac vessels. The duodenum is partly seen surrounding the pancreas and may contain dense oral contrast. The kidneys and adrenal glands are partly seen.

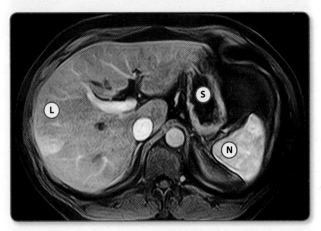

Figure 2.17 Axial T1-weighted post-contrast MRI at T11 level shows bright signal in the blood vessels. Ⓢ stomach, Ⓛ liver, Ⓝ spleen are well visualised.

T1-weighted MR images display mesenteric fat as bright signal. The liver is seen with homogeneous signal and appears slightly more hyperintense than the spleen. The gallbladder appears of low signal. All blood vessels are dark due to flow voids (**Figure 2.18**).

Midabdomen

At this level (L3 vertebra), small intestinal loops and colon fill the abdominal cavity. Both the kidneys are

Clinical insight

- Cross-sectional images (US, CT and MRI) are presented as if looking at the patient 'through the feet'. Therefore the right side of the body is on the left of image (**Figure 2.19**)
- Coronal images are oriented as if the body is facing the viewer, and again the right side of the body is on the left of the image (**Figure 2.20**)
- Sagittal views are presented with the patient facing towards the left of the image, so the spine is towards the right whereas the front of the abdomen is towards the left of the image (**Figure 2.21**)

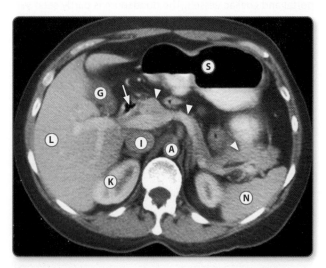

Figure 2.18 Axial CT image at transpyloric plane. Ⓛ Liver; Ⓖ Gallbladder; Ⓢ Stomach; Ⓝ Spleen; Ⓚ right kidney. Duodenum (arrow) is seen around the pancreas (arrowheads). Portal vein courses posterior to the pancreas and is denser than the pancreatic tissue. The aorta Ⓐ is surrounded by the diaphragmatic crura.

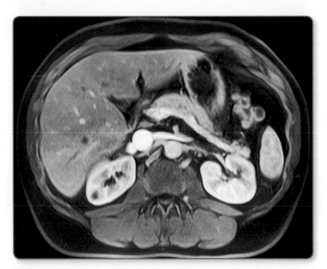

Figure 2.19 Axial T1-weighted post-contrast MRI just below transpyloric plane shows bright signal in the blood vessels. The liver, spleen and pancreas are well visualised. The left renal hilum displays the renal vein.

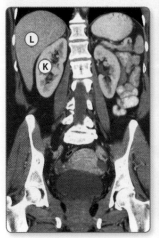

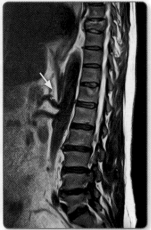

Figure 2.20 Coronal CT scan shows the spine, (K) kidneys and (L) liver. Note that patient's right side is on the left of the image.

Figure 2.21 Sagittal MRI with the spine on the right side of the image. The coeliac artery is seen arising from the aorta (arrow).

seen at this level along with renal vessels and the ureters (**Figure 2.22**).

Pelvis

On axial images:

- The pelvic wall is seen, made up of the iliac bones and the psoas and iliacus muscles (**Figures 2.23** and **2.24**).
- The bladder is visualised as a fluid-filled structure (**Figures 2.23** and **2.24**).
- The uterus (**Figure 2.23**) lies between the bladder and rectum in women.
- The ovaries may also be seen connected to the uterus by the fallopian tubes (**Figure 2.23**).
- The ascending and descending colon are seen in both flanks as tubular structures.

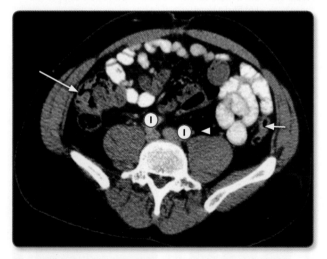

Figure 2.22 Axial CT at L3 level showing bowel loops in the abdomen. Ascending (long arrow) and descending colon (short arrow) are seen in right and left flanks respectively. Left ureter (arrowhead) is seen adjacent to the iliac vessels ⓘ.

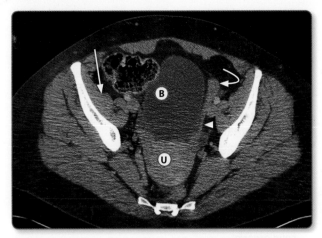

Figure 2.23 Axial CT scan of the midpelvis showing the dense iliac bones on either side. Psoas and iliacus muscles (arrow) line the inside of the pelvic cavity. Mottled densities are seen in the caecum containing gas and faecal matter. (**B**) bladder appearing as a fluid-filled structure; (**U**) uterus posterior to the bladder. The left ovary (curved arrow) is seen attached to the uterus by fallopian tube (arrowhead)

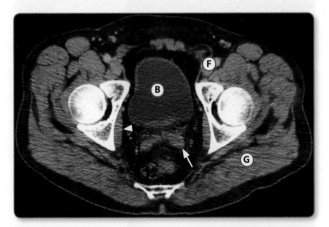

Figure 2.24 Axial CT of the pelvis at level of hip joints. (**B**) bladder, again seen as a fluid-filled structure. The obturator internus muscle lines the pelvis at this level (arrowhead). The seminal vesicles appear as triangular structures below the bladder (arrow). (**F**) femoral vessels, (**G**) gluteus muscle

T2-weighted MR images display bright signal in the fluid-filled urinary bladder and gallbladder (**Figure 2.25**). T1-weighted images display mesenteric fat as bright signal and allow easy distinction of solid organs, hollow organs and muscles. MRI may also be used to study the biliary tract and this examination is called MR cholangiopancreatography (MRCP) (**Figure 2.26**).

Step-by-step approach to interpreting cross-sectional images

1. Identify the organ being examined
2. Identify the normal density or signal intensity of the organ, e.g. liver and spleen are homogeneous, whereas the kidney shows different densities in its cortex and medulla
3. Identify if any hypo- or hyperdense areas are present in the solid organs

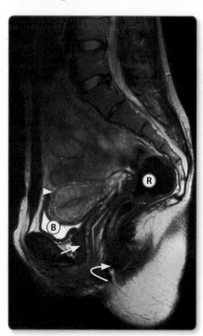

Figure 2.25 Sagittal T2-weighted MRI in the midline showing the uterus (arrowhead). Muscular elements in the urethral complex (arrow) and anal canal (curved arrow) have a darker signal. Ⓑ bladder, Ⓡ rectum; solid line, vagina. Note that images of the bowel are blurred because of respiratory and peristaltic movements.

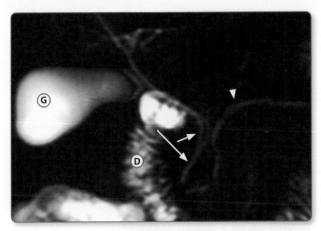

Figure 2.26 MR cholangiopancreatography examination showing the pancreatic duct (arrowhead), common bile duct (arrow) and cystic duct (short arrow) joining the common bile duct. Ⓖ gallbladder, Ⓓ duodenum.

4. Identify if any abnormal densities (calcification) are present in the organs
5. Identify if any fluid (0 HU) is present in the abdomen surrounding the organs
6. Identify if any of the psoas margins or peritoneal flanks are obscured by fluid or inflammation
7. Identify any abnormal opacity in the mesenteric fat
8. Identify any abnormal bowel distension
9. Identify the major vessels (aorta, inferior vena cava) and assess if there are any filling defects or calcification in the arteries
10. Identify if any fluid-containing haemorrhage (>100 HU) is present in cysts, organs or the abdominal cavity.

2.5 CT angiography

CT angiography (CTA) is a non-invasive screening technique used for detection of GI tract bleeding and mesenteric ischaemia (**Figure 2.27**). CTA allows faster acquisition times (compared with catheter angiography), allowing assessment

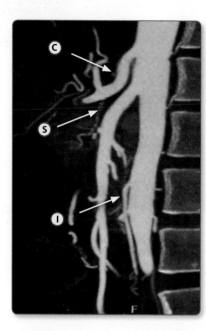

Figure 2.27 CT angiography examination showing the aorta and mesenteric vessels. (S) superior mesenteric artery, (I) inferior mesenteric artery (C) coeliac.

of visceral branches and the mesenteric arteries. Scanning is done while injection of contrast is at a high flow rate (4 ml/s) through an antecubital vein. Images are acquired while the contrast is in the arterial circulation (at approximately 20–30 s). Images may also be acquired at a slightly later time (50–60 s) to obtain images of the venous system.

chapter 3

Recognising abnormalities

3.1 Fat-line abnormalities

Abnormalities of fat lines and stripes can provide valuable information about the underlying pathology. However, it must be noted that fat stripes may normally be absent, particularly in children, due to deficient

> **Clinical insight**
>
> Abnormalities of fat lines, lymph nodes or mesenteric streaking often point to underlying pathology nearby. Thorough evaluation of adjacent organs often results in diagnosis of the condition.

mesenteric fat. The right psoas margin may be absent in up to 20% of adult patients, so care must be taken not to place undue emphasis solely on abnormalities of fat stripes.

Definition

The abnormalities are visualisation of normal fat density lines on the radiograph.

Pathophysiology

When normal mesenteric or peritoneal fat is infiltrated with inflammatory exudate or oedema, it loses its normal density and becomes similar in density to solid organs, resulting in blurring or complete loss of visualisation against the normal organs.

Examples

- Loss of the normal fat stripes may be commonly seen in intra-abdominal inflammatory conditions
- Inflammatory conditions in the right iliac fossa such as acute appendicitis may cause loss of the peritoneal fat line and obliteration of the lower right psoas margin (**Figure 3.1**)
- The renal margins may be obscured in inflammatory conditions such as pyelonephritis

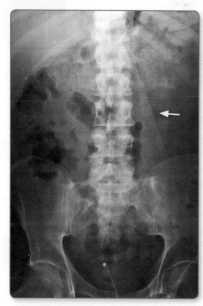

Figure 3.1 Radiograph showing obscuration of the right psoas margin in a patient with appendicitis. Arrow is the left psoas margin.

- Pancreatitis causes loss of the psoas margins on both sides
- Left-sided diverticulitis may cause obscuration of the left lower peritoneal fat stripe (**Figure 3.2**)
- On CT and MRI, inflammation involving solid organs or the bowel causes streaking of the adjacent fat in the mesentery and blurring of the margins of affected organs, due to oedema and inflammatory exudates blurring the interface between the normal fat and solid tissues (**Figure 3.3**)

3.2 Gas shadow abnormalities

Definition

These abnormalities are abnormal location of gas shadows, gas shadows in abnormal orientations and large collections of gas within a distended viscus.

Pathophysiology

- Gas may be outside the bowel lumen due to perforation or fistulation

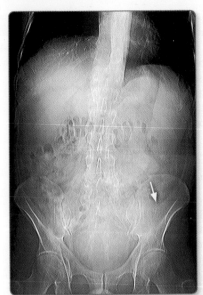

Figure 3.2 Abdominal radiograph showing abrupt loss of the left peritoneal fat stripe (arrow) in a patient with sigmoid diverticulitis.

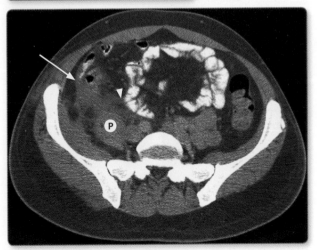

Figure 3.3 CT image showing marked inflammation around the appendix that blurs tissue margins (arrow). Note inflammation obliterates fat lines laterally and along psoas margins (P). Normal mesenteric fat is seen along the left psoas muscle.

- Obstruction of the bowel can cause dilatation of the lumen with gas
- Gas in abnormal places such as bile ducts or abscesses may have an abnormal orientation and not follow normal bowel contours

> ## Guiding principle
>
> Free air in the peritoneal cavity produces several distinct radiological signs, such as:
>
> - gas under the diaphragm
> - Rigler's sign
> - football sign
> - falciform ligament sign

Examples

Abnormal location

- Bowel perforation allows gas to collect in the peritoneal cavity, often seen on chest radiographs as a curvilinear area of lucency under the diaphragm
- Rigler's sign (**Figure 3.4**) shows gas both inside and outside the bowel with a sharp margin of the bowel wall
- Free gas can also outline abnormal ligaments, such as the curvilinear shadow lateral to the upper lumbar vertebra on the right (**falciform ligament sign – Figure 3.5**)

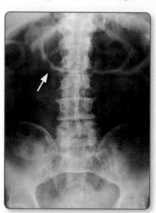

Figure 3.4 Radiograph showing Rigler's sign around the transverse colon (arrow).

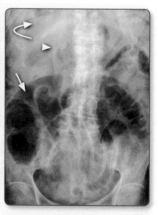

Figure 3.5 Radiograph showing pneumoperitoneum outlining the falciform ligament (arrowhead) and forming triangular pockets within mesenteric leaves (arrow). Note air lucency over the liver (curved arrow).

- Lots of air in the peritoneal cavity creates a uniform, ovoid lucency over the entire abdomen in the shape of an American football (the 'football' or 'dome' sign)
- Occasionally air can also be seen within the bile ducts or the portal vein, the former secondary to sphincterotomy or gallstone fistulation (**Figure 3.6**) and the latter seen in bowel infarction or necrotising enterocolitis

Abnormal orientation

- Gas within abscesses may also lie outside the normal configuration of the bowel, with a mottled appearance and, if large, may show a fluid level
- Free gas within the *mesentery* creates triangular shadows between the mesenteric leaves and bowel wall (see **Figure 3.5**)
- Excessive amounts of gas and fluid within an obstructed intestinal segment create multiple fluid levels, especially on an erect radiograph

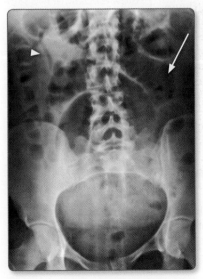

Figure 3.6 Radiograph showing bowel dilatation (arrow) and pneumobilia (arrowhead).

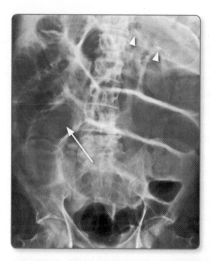

Figure 3.7 Radiograph showing small bowel obstruction with dilated loops exceeding 3 cm in diameter (arrow). Note calcification in pancreas across the midline (arrowheads).

Abnormal distension

- Small bowel distension exceeding 3 cm is indicative of obstruction (**Figure 3.7**). This is gas normally present within the bowel which, due to obstruction, accumulates and creates distension

> **Clinical insight**
>
> In a normal adult, the height of a lumbar vertebra varies between 3 and 3.5 cm, so any small bowel loop that is wider than the lumbar vertebra is abnormally distended.

- Large bowel is more distensible and obstruction is indicated by a distension >5 cm
- Obstructed bowel segments with lots of fluid can show the 'string of pearls' sign, because tiny bubbles of gas outline the segment

3.3 Calcifications

Definition

Abdominal calcifications are dense opacities projected on radiographs or CT scans.

Pathophysiology

- Most abnormal abdominal calcifications are non-visceral and occur in mesenteric nodes and blood vessels; they are dystrophic in type and occur in areas of damaged or degenerating tissue or hyalinised scars in blood vessels
- Calcific opacities related to specific organs may provide a clue to the underlying clinical condition such as calculi or specific tumours
- Calcification also occurs in areas of stasis, leading to stone formation, e.g. kidney, gallbladder, urinary bladder and bowel diverticula

Examples

Renal calculi Dense, calcified opacities may be seen overlying the renal shadow on radiographs in patients with renal colic (**Figure 3.8**). Large calculi may have a staghorn configuration. Ureteric calculi lie along the line of the ureter, which is along the tips of the transverse processes of the vertebral bodies.

Gallstones Most gallstones are not visualised on radiographs; approximately 10% typically appear as small faceted opacities. Curvilinear calcification of the gallbladder wall leads to a porcelain gallbladder appearance.

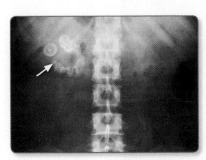

Figure 3.8 Radiograph showing multiple renal calculi in the left kidney (arrow).

Enteroliths Occasionally faceted or large stones may be seen in the lower abdomen or right iliac fossa. These are likely to be appendicoliths or enteroliths (concretion or calculus within the gastrointestinal tract particularly in areas of stasis) within Meckel's diverticulum (**Figure 3.9**).

Pancreatic Calcification may be seen in the pancreas, which is typically specular (spotty with specks of calcification) and seen along the transpyloric plane. Calcification of the pancreas occurs in the setting of chronic pancreatitis due to dystrophic calcification in areas of degeneration and necrosis (see **Figure 3.7**).

Aneurysmal Calcification is often seen in the abdominal aorta or aortic aneurysms.

Tumoral Calcified teeth or bones may be seen in large dermoid tumours in the abdomen or pelvis (**Figure 3.10**). Faint stippled calcification may be seen in renal cell carcinomas, neuroblastomas and certain liver tumours.

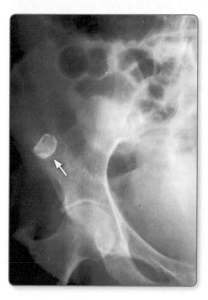

Figure 3.9 Radiograph showing a large enterolith (arrow) in the right iliac fossa. This was within Meckel's diverticulum.

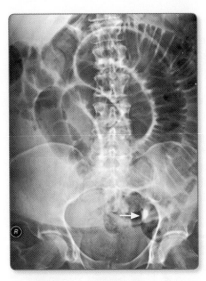

Figure 3.10 Radiograph showing a large tooth-shaped calcification (arrow) in the pelvis with the associated mass effect displacing bowel loops. This was calcification in a large dermoid cyst.

3.4 Abnormalities on barium examinations

Definition

Abnormalities on barium examination may be related to filling defects secondary to mass lesions, mucosal abnormalities secondary to inflammation or ulceration, or abnormalities of peristalsis.

Pathophysiology

- Large mass lesions appear as filling defects within the barium column
- Inflammation or infiltration of the intestinal mucosal folds leads to thickening or nodularity
- Ulcer craters contain a speck of barium surrounded by a ring of oedema and create a 'target pattern lesion'

Examples

Filling defects These are typically formed by mass lesions projecting within the bowel lumen (**Figure 3.11**). Unusually foreign bodies or even parasitic infections can cause filling defects (**Figure 3.12**), and a circumferential filling defect such as that caused by an annular cancer leads to the 'apple-core' appearance of colorectal cancer.

Ulceration Ulcers appear as target lesions or linear out-pouching or tracks of barium outside the bowel lumen. The former occur when a small amount of barium in an ulcer crater is surrounded by an elevated, oedematous, ulcer mound. When seen in profile, deep ulcers are outlined by

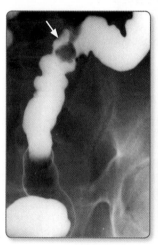

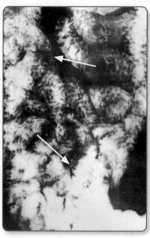

Figure 3.11 Barium examination showing a filling defect caused by a pedunculated polyp in the sigmoid colon (arrow).

Figure 3.12 Filling defects on barium examinations are usually caused by tumours. However, in this case the linear filling defects (arrows) are caused by roundworms (*Ascaris lumbricoides*).

barium and appear as linear tracks or spiculations arising from the bowel lumen. Deep ulcers may be seen in Crohn's disease and superficial ulcers are seen in ulcerative colitis, peptic ulcers and certain infections.

Mucosal fold abnormalities Diffuse infiltration of the intestinal wall due to inflammation or infection can cause fold thickening and distortion. Thickening of the mucosal folds is seen in intestinal infections, and nodular folds are seen in lymphoma. Reversal of the fold pattern in the jejunum and ileum is seen in coeliac disease, and diffuse granularity of the mucosa and loss of haustral pattern are seen in ulcerative colitis (lead-pipe colon).

3.5 Solid organ abnormalities

Definition
Abnormalities involving solid organs may be due to changes in size, contour, and different X-ray attenuation, or contrast enhancement on cross-sectional examination such as US, CT or MRI.

Pathophysiology
Abdominal organs may be enlarged in size due to pathological changes or malignant infiltration, pathological changes or lesions possibly having different attenuation values on cross-sectional examinations. Furthermore, these lesions may have different enhancement patterns compared with intrinsic normal organs.

Examples

Difference in attenuation or signal intensity
Liver metastases typically have reduced enhancement compared with the normal hepatic parenchyma, therefore appearing as hypointense or hypodense rounded shadows on MRI

and CT respectively (**Figure 3.13**). This is because most metastases are supplied by the hepatic artery (which supplies the hepatic interstitium where metastases occur) rather than the portal vein, the latter generally supplying the liver parenchyma and hepatocytes.

Therefore, due to the larger blood supply of the portal vein, metastases appear less vascular. Larger metastases also appear hypodense as they outgrow their blood supply.

Enlargement in size or contour

- Inflamed or diseased organs may increase in size due to oedema, increased cellular infiltrates or tumour involvement (**Figures 3.14** and **3.15**)

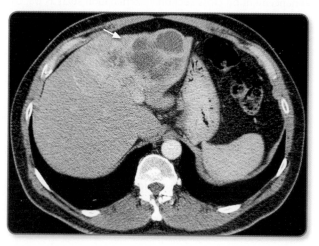

Figure 3.13 CT scan showing a hypodense lesion in the liver (arrow) caused by colon cancer metastases.

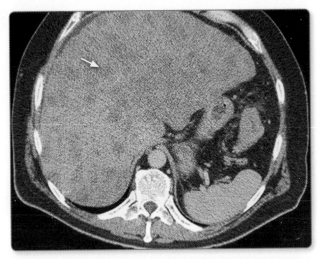

Figure 3.14 CT scan showing enlargement of the liver due to diffuse infiltration and involvement with metastatic disease (arrow).

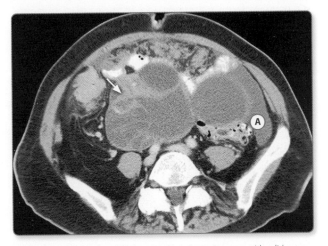

Figure 3.15 CT scan showing a large multicystic ovarian mass with solid elements (arrow) and ascites (A).

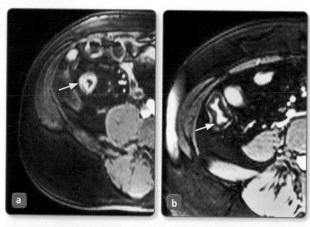

Figure 3.16 Abnormalities in bowel pattern. MR images show (a) Target sign in bowel inflammation (arrow) due to enhancing inner and outer rings (mucosa and serosa) and isodense submucosa in the middle. (b) Halo sign of chronic bowel inflammation caused by a dark submucosal layer (arrow) secondary to fibrosis.

- Inflamed bowel in Crohn's disease becomes thickened and oedematous and usually measures >3 mm in wall thickness (**Figure 3.16**)
- Cirrhotic liver demonstrates contour changes and typically has a nodular or bumpy outline
- Blurring of organ margins and adjacent mesenteric fat is another sign of underlying pathology (see **Figure 3.3**).

Gastrointestinal system

The gastrointestinal (GI) system consists of the GI tract, a muscular tube from the oesophagus to the anal canal, which has the primary role of digestion of food and expulsion of waste matter as faeces. The small intestine is up to 7 metres (5 m on average), whereas the large intestine is about 1.5 m in length. Important conditions affecting the GI tract are colorectal cancers, bowel obstruction and ulceration. Acute conditions such as bowel obstruction form a significant percentage of acute admissions to the accident and emergency department (A & E). CT examinations remain the mainstay of GI tract imaging in the acute setting. MRI is used in the staging of rectal cancers and in inflammatory bowel disease. Barium examinations are mainly used for assessment of the mucosa and fold pattern of the bowel, which provide diagnostic information about underlying pathology.

4.1 Achalasia

Achalasia is a rare motility disorder of the oesophagus, with an incidence of approximately 1 in 100,000. It is caused by the absence of or damage to the nervous system of the oesophagus (Auerbach's plexus). The clinical symptoms are insidious and usually present in the fourth to fifth decades. The most common symptom is dysphagia (difficulty in swallowing). Odynophagia (chest pain on swallowing) may be a prominent symptom in some patients.

Key facts

- There is an absence of both oesophageal peristalsis and relaxation of the lower oesophageal sphincter (LES) after swallowing

- Sphincter constriction creates an obstruction, increasing pressure in the proximal oesophagus and causing it to progressively dilate
- Aspiration of oesophageal contents can result in risk of lung abscesses and pneumonia.

Radiological findings

Chest radiograph A widened mediastinum and an air–fluid level may be seen (**Figure 4.1**) because obstruction at the gastro-oesophageal junction causes accumulation of food matter and fluid in the dilated upper oesophagus. A dilated oesophagus creates a widened mediastinum whereas food debris creates an air–fluid level.

Barium swallow examination As the gastro-oesophageal sphincter does not relax normally, barium does not pass into the stomach. Swallowed barium remains in the oesophagus until the hydrostatic pressure exerted by the fluid column overcomes the resistance of the sphincter. Barium then dribbles and squirts

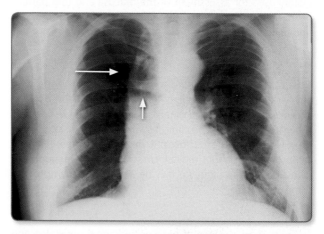

Figure 4.1 Chest radiograph showing widened mediastinum (long arrow) with air–fluid lucency (short arrow) in a patient with achalasia. Note absence of air in the gastric fundus

through a narrow opening into the stomach. The oesophagus is markedly dilated (>4 cm). The head of the barium column as it passes through the sphincter forms an elongated 'V'-shaped configuration likened to a bird's beak (**Figure 4.2**).

Key imaging findings

A. Dilated oesophagus from accumulation of food matter and fluid
B. A widened mediastinum from the dilated oesophagus
C. Air–fluid level from accumulation of food and fluid
D. 'Bird-beak' appearance of the gastro-oesophageal junction.

Treatment

Usually, a lengthwise cut of the outer muscle layers of the LES (Heller's myotomy) can help (approximately 90%). Other procedures, such as radiological or endoscopic balloon dilatation of the LES, can also be used.

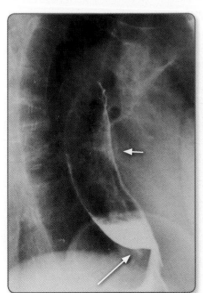

Figure 4.2 Barium swallow examination shows a dilated oesophagus (short arrow) with a tapered, narrow opening at the gastro-esophageal junction (long arrow) creating a bird-beak appearance

4.2 Appendicitis

Appendicitis is an acute inflammation of the vermiform appendix. It is the most common acute abdominal condition in children. Patients typically present with pain over McBurney's point (point one third of the distance on a line joining the anterosuperior iliac spine to the umbilicus). Nausea, diarrhoea, fever and vomiting may also be present. The incidence of appendicitis is approximately 1 per 1000 and the peak incidence is in the late teenage years.

Key facts

- Appendicitis is caused by obstruction of the appendiceal lumen due to appendicoliths, mucus plugs or rarely tumours
- Non-specific symptoms may delay diagnosis, which leads to a higher appendiceal perforation rate
- Perforation may lead to abdominal abscess formation.

Radiological findings

Radiograph Non-specific, but may demonstrate localised ileus (distended bowel loops) in the right iliac fossa and calcified appendicoliths (**Figure 4.3**).

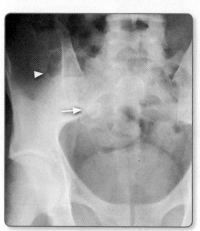

Figure 4.3 Radiograph showing a calcified appendicolith (arrow). Note localised small bowel ileus with fluid levels (arrowhead).

US US plays an important role in the diagnosis of acute appendicitis, because the appendix can be directly visualised to confirm or exclude appendiceal pathology. The inflamed appendix is seen as a thickened, non-compressible, tubular structure at the site of tenderness measuring >6 mm in diameter (**Figure 4.4**). A diameter of >6 mm has a high positive predictive value in the diagnosis of appendicitis (>95%). An echogenic appendicolith may be seen in up to 30% of cases and enlarged mesenteric nodes are often present. Patients with appendiceal perforation may present with a right iliac fossa mass, which typically consists of the inflamed appendix with adherent omental and mesenteric fat – termed an 'appendiceal phlegmon'. CT may be used in patients with equivocal US results or in heavier patients in whom a US examination may be technically difficult.

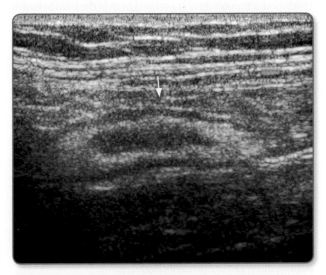

Figure 4.4 US showing a distended tubular structure in the right iliac fossa (arrow). Inflammatory changes and mesenteric oedema are seen as hypoechoic areas behind the appendix

Key imaging findings
A. Thickened tubular struc-
ture in the right iliac fossa
B. Appendicolith
C. Diameter >6 mm
D. Non-compressible
appendix

Treatment
Surgical appendicectomy.

4.3 Coeliac disease

Coeliac disease, also known as non-tropical sprue, is the most
common intestinal disorder causing malabsorption. The average incidence is 1 in 100 people. Patients usually present in
childhood, although there is a second peak in the third to fourth
decades. The classic presentation is with steatorrhoea, weight
loss and failure to thrive.

Key facts
- It is caused by intestinal hypersensitivity to gluten in food
- The main complications of chronic coeliac disease are development of intestinal lymphoma and carcinoma of the
oesophagus
- Extensive ulcerative jejunoileitis is another rare complication.

Radiological findings

Barium examination The classic sign is the 'reversed jejunoileal pattern', in which the ileum demonstrates more mucosal
folds than usual, whereas there is a reduced number of folds
of the jejunum (**Figure 4.5**). This causes a reversal of the fold
pattern observed in normal individuals.

The progressive loss of mucosal folds in the jejunum gives it a
colonic appearance in advanced cases. The 'Moulage sign' is seen
in advanced cases where no mucosal folds are seen and the entire

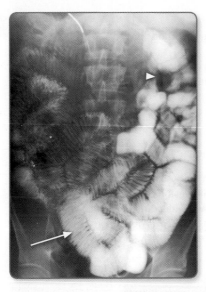

Figure 4.5 Enteroclysis examination shows closely packed mucosal folds (jejunal pattern) in the ileum – 'reversal sign' (arrow). Clumping of barium and colonic appearance of jejunum is also present (arrowhead).

intestine appears as a featureless tube. Hypersecretion and excessive fluid in the intestine cause dilution and clumping of barium.

Key imaging findings
A. Reversed jejunoileal pattern
B. Colonic appearance of jejunum
C. Moulage sign
D. Clumping of barium

Treatment

Restriction and avoidance of gluten in diet.

4.4 Colorectal cancer

Colorectal cancer arises from the mucosa of the colon and typically has a polypoid appearance.

Most cancers are adenocarcinomas (98%), the most common cancers of the GI tract. Rectal bleeding, weight loss and change in bowel habits are common presenting symptoms. Anaemia may be a predominant symptom in right-sided colon cancers.

Key facts

- Most patients have mutations in the *K-RAS*, *APC*, *p53* and *DCC* genes
- A small proportion of colorectal cancers is associated with polyposis syndromes and pre-existing inflammatory bowel disease
- Large cancers may cause complications such as bowel obstruction.

Radiological findings

Barium examination Early cancers may be seen as small polypoid or plaque-like lesions. Polypoid lesions may have an irregular contour with ulcerations, and larger lesions or circumferential lesions produce an 'apple-core' stricture (**Figure 4.6**). The affected segment typically shows rigidity with loss of normal peristalsis.

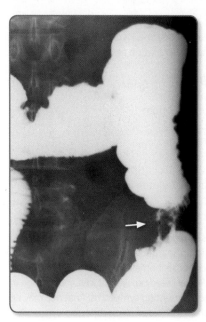

Figure 4.6 Barium enema examination showing a concentric narrowing of the descending colon due to tumour. This appearance is termed an 'apple-core stricture' (arrow).

CT CT is the predominant modality used for staging colorectal cancer. Cancers appear as areas of irregular thickening of the colonic wall with an intraluminal mass. Extension into the pericolic fat and lymphadenopathy may be present (**Figure 4.7**). Distant metastases to the liver or lungs may be present in advanced cancers.

MRI This plays a key role in the staging of rectal cancers because accurate TNM (tumour, node, metastasis) staging is needed before total mesorectal excision. With its high contrast sensitivity, MRI can differentiate between advanced and localised tumours (**Figure 4.8**). This is critical because advanced tumours (≥T3 or >N1) require chemo-/radiotherapy before surgery. T3 tumours are seen as extensions of the primary tumour into the surrounding mesorectal fat. (MRI is not used for staging other colonic cancers because normal respiratory motions make it difficult to obtain optimal images. The rectum, being retroperitoneal, does not move with respiration and therefore can be imaged without any movement artefacts).

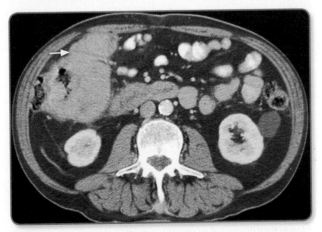

Figure 4.7 Axial CT scan of the abdomen showing a large hepatic flexure tumour (arrow). The tumour invades into the mesocolic fat and anteriorly involves the peritoneum and anterior abdominal wall muscles.

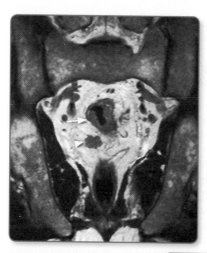

Figure 4.8 Coronal T2-weighted MR scan showing rectal tumour (arrow) extending into the mesorectal fat. Note enlarged lymph node (arrowhead).

Key imaging findings

A. Polypoid lesions, on barium examination, >2 cm
B. Fixity and infiltration of the affected bowel segment
C. Ulceration
D. Apple-core stricture

Treatment

Treatment of colon cancers is with total surgical resection with or without pre-/post-surgical chemotherapy and radiotherapy.

Clinical insight

Current generation multidetector CT scanners can obtain virtual images of the entire colon (**Figure 4.9**). This is called a CT colonographic examination and is reported to have similar accuracy to colonoscopy without its attendant complications. Studies have shown that screening for polyps or cancers can be provided with a CT colonography examination.

4.5 Diverticulitis

Diverticula are acquired herniations of colonic mucosa through the muscular layer and such a condition is termed 'diverticulosis'. Inflammation of colonic diverticula is termed 'diverticulitis'. Acute diverticulitis is a common cause of large bowel obstruction. Patients may present with colicky pain, raised white blood cell counts, fever, malaise, pain and palpable masses.

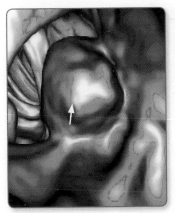

Figure 4.9 Virtual endoscopic view from a CT colonogram study showing a large polypoid cancer (arrow).

Key facts

- Diverticulosis is the most common colonic disease in the world and diverticulitis is its most common presentation
- Inflammation of the diverticula may lead to localised perforations and abscess formation.

Radiological findings

US Pericolic inflammation is seen as an area of increased echogenicity and abscesses appear as hypoechoic rounded areas. Often an echogenic faecolith (inspissated organic matter and food debris) is seen within the inflamed area. Maximum tenderness can be elicited by compression at the site of the abnormal findings.

CT This is the best modality for assessment and diagnosis of diverticulitis (sensitivity >90%). Diverticulitis appears as an area of colonic wall thickening with streaking of adjacent pericolic fat (**Figure 4.10**). Air-containing diverticula may be observed within the area of inflammation. Localised abscesses appear as hypodense collections (**Figure 4.11**). The 'arrowhead sign' may also be seen, a result of increased enhancement and oedema at the orifice of the inflamed diverticulum.

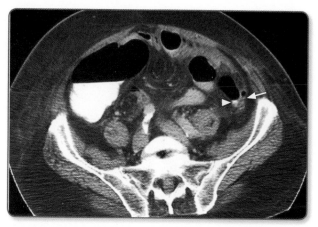

Figure 4.10 CT scan of the abdomen showing inflamed diverticulum with pericolic inflammation (arrow). Dense contrast at orifice of diverticulum (arrowhead).

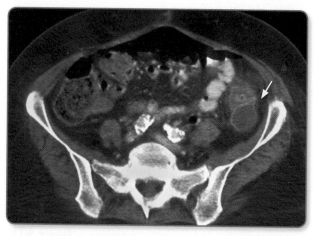

Figure 4.11 CT scan of the abdomen showing a small abscess adjacent to inflamed diverticulum (arrow).

Key imaging findings
A. Pericolic inflammation
B. Faecoliths
C. Colonic thickening with streaky changes in the mesocolon
D. Arrowhead sign.

Treatment

Treatment is usually by antibiotic therapy. Abscesses may need to be drained percutaneously under radiological guidance.

4.6 Gastric cancer

Most gastric cancers are adenocarcinomas (95%) and they arise from the gastric mucosa. Patients may present with weight loss, anaemia, anorexia or melaena, although an advanced, even a metastatic stage can be symptomless. Virchow's node – a hard, swollen, left supraclavicular lymph node – is a classic presentation of gastric cancer.

Key facts

- Environmental factors play a significant role in the development of gastric cancer
- Patients with pernicious anaemia are 20 times more likely to develop cancer
- High consumption of salted or smoked foods and *Helicobacter pylori* (*H. pylori*) infections are other predisposing factors

Radiological findings

Barium examination Gastric cancer has three distinct radiological appearances:
1. Most cases are ulcerative lesions. Malignant ulcers typically have thick everted edges and an irregular contour (**Figure 4.12**). There may be associated mass or irregular radiating folds around the ulcer
2. Polypoid lesion (10%)
3. Scirrhous type (10%) in which there is marked desmoplastic

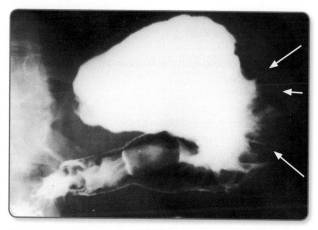

Figure 4.12 Barium examination showing a stomach cancer involving the greater curvature with irregular penetrating ulcers (arrows).

reaction (growth of dense fibrous tissue around the tumour) and thickening of the gastric wall. This type is frequently referred to as linitis plastica and is uniformly fatal. Linitis plastica appears as a contracted stomach with loss of the normal rugal folds.

CT This used for staging of gastric cancer. Cancer appears as irregular thickening (>1.5 cm) of the gastric wall or polypoid lesions. Linitis plastica is seen as diffuse thickening of the entire stomach (**Figure 4.13**). Adjacent infiltration of the pancreas or retroperitoneum may be easily detected on CT scans. In recent years positron emission tomography (PET)-CT has also been employed in staging of gastric and oesophageal tumours, because it has greater sensitivity for detecting pathological lymphadenopathy than CT.

Key imaging findings

A. Malignant ulcer
B. Polypoid mass
C. Contracted stomach with loss of rugae (linitis plastica)
D. Thickening of the gastric wall >15 mm.

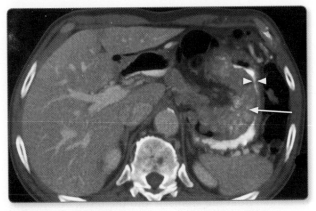

Figure 4.13 CT scan of a gastric cancer showing marked thickening of the stomach wall (arrow) and contraction of the lumen (arrowheads).

Treatment
Surgical gastrectomy. Radiotherapy or chemotherapy may also be used.

4.7 Gastro-oesophageal reflux disease

Gastro-oesophageal reflux disease (GERD) is the most common abnormality of the oesophagus. The common symptoms associated with GERD are heartburn, chest pain and dysphagia.

Key facts
- A hiatus hernia is present in most patients with GERD, which, by chronically irritating the oesophageal epithelium, can lead to chronic oesophagitis; this in turn may lead to Barrett's oesophagus – a change in the oesophageal epithelium of squamous to columnar cells
- Barrett's oesophagus, similar to other chronic inflammation-induced metaplasias, predisposes to cancer formation (more than 30 times that in the normal population) and is associated with oesophageal strictures.

Radiological findings

Barium examination These remain the primary radiological modality in the examination of GERD. Hiatus hernias are of two types: an axial type that is seen as a small portion of stomach herniating above the diaphragm into the thorax (**Figure 4.14**), and a para-oesophageal type that is seen as a small loculus of stomach herniating behind the oesophagus, although the gastro-oesophageal junction remains below the diaphragm.

Oesophagitis is seen as thickened folds (>3 mm) in the distal oesophagus. Small ulcers may be present. On positional manoeuvres and Valsalva's manoeuvre there is reflux of barium from the stomach into the distal oesophagus (**Figure 4.15**). In Barrett's oesophagus deep ulcers may be seen along with ring-like strictures in the mid- to distal oesophagus.

Key imaging findings
A. Hiatus hernia
B. Thickened folds and ulcers

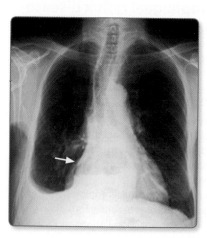

Figure 4.14 Chest radiograph showing a large hiatus hernia as a gas-filled structure (arrow) in the lower mediastinum.

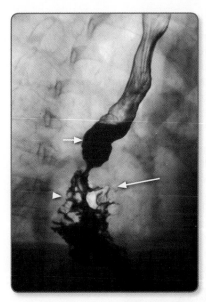

Figure 4.15 Barium swallow examination showing a fixed hernia above the diaphragm (long arrow) with thickened mucosal folds (arrowhead) and reflux of barium into the lower oesophagus (short arrow).

C. Strictures
D. Reflux of barium into distal oesophagus.

Treatment

Antacids and a reduction in alcohol consumption and smoking usually provide adequate treatment.

4.8 GI tract haemorrhage

GI haemorrhage can be classified into upper or lower GI bleeds. The most common causes for upper GI bleeds are gastric erosions (20%), duodenal ulcers (30%) and gastro-oesophageal varices (30%). An acute lower GI bleed is less common and can be caused by diverticulosis or angiodysplasias (vascular malformation). Most diverticular bleeds are right sided; this is because right-sided diverticula have wider necks and domes, which exposes the blood vessel stretched over them to injury and perforation.

Key facts

- Most acute upper and lower GI bleeds are investigated using endoscopy or colonoscopy
- Radiology plays a part if these investigations are negative and bleeding from the small intestine is suspected, especially in cases with slow or intermittent GI bleeds.

Radiological findings

Angiography/CT Angiography is performed by selective catheterisation of the coeliac and mesenteric arteries. Bleeding is seen as focal areas of contrast extravasation from the arteries (**Figure 4.16**). Causative factors such as aneurysms or vascular malformations may also be demonstrated. CT angiography (CTA) is a useful triaging tool for diagnosing or excluding active GI haemorrhage, localising the site of bleeding and guiding subsequent treatment. Contrast extravasation may be seen at point of bleeding on CT scans (**Figure 4.17**). The advantages

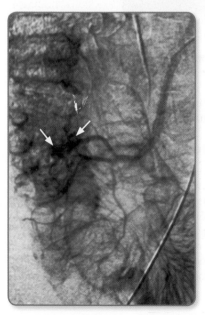

Figure 4.16 Mesenteric angiogram shows extravasation of contrast (bleeding) as small dense pools (arrows) in the ascending colon.

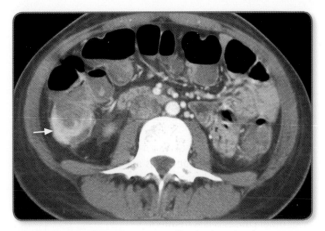

Figure 4.17 CT angiogram showing active bleeding (arrow) as dense spots within the right colonic lumen.

are that CTA is non-invasive and allows detection of both arterial and venous bleeding sites, whereas catheter angiography allows detection of only arterial bleeds.

Nuclear scans ^{99m}Tc-tagged red blood cell (RBC) scanning is the most sensitive technique for detection of active GI bleeding and allows imaging over a prolonged period, making it useful also for detecting intermittent bleeding. Tagged RBCs accumulate by extravasation at the site of the bleed and appear as hot spots on nuclear imaging.

Key imaging findings
A. Extravasation of contrast on angiography
B. Hyperdense contrast extravasation from arteries or veins on CTA
C. Associated aneurysms or vascular malformations
D. Hot spots on tagged RBC nuclear imaging.

Treatment
Surgical excision of the causative agent or radiological transcatheter embolisation of bleeding point.

4.9 Ischaemic colitis

Ischaemic colitis is a condition in which there is sudden inflammation of part of the colon due to loss of or reduction in blood flow to that segment. Ischaemic colitis is the most common vascular disorder of the GI tract in patients aged >65 years. Patients usually present with sudden, severe, abdominal pain, tenesmus and bloody diarrhoea.

Key facts

- Most cases of ischaemic colitis are due to vascular hypoperfusion as a result of arteriosclerosis, vasogenic shock or cardiac conditions
- Ischaemia due to vascular occlusion by thrombus, emboli or other causes is less frequent
- The most commonly affected site is the splenic flexure, followed by the descending and sigmoid colon.

Radiological findings

Radiograph 'Thumb-printing' of the colon (**Figure 4.18**) is seen

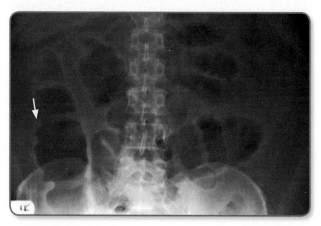

Figure 4.18 Radiograph showing thumbprinting (arrow) of the colon in a patient with ischaemic colitis.

as small indentations on the colonic wall caused by submucosal oedema. The colon may also appear distended. Pneumatosis coli (air within the bowel wall) may be observed and in advanced cases there may be perforation with signs of pneumoperitoneum (free air within the abdominal cavity) (**Figure 4.19**).

US The findings include segmental or circumferential colonic wall thickening, pericolic changes, reduced or absent peristalsis, and diminished blood flow on Doppler studies.

CT This shows colonic thickening, ascites and absence of normal enhancement of the affected segment. Marked oedema of the bowel is present and embolic clots may block the mesenteric vessels.

Key imaging findings
A. Thumb printing
B. Pneumatosis
C. Lack of blood flow on Doppler studies
D. Clots in mesenteric arteries.

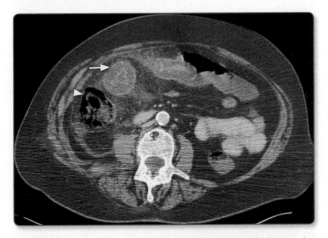

Figure 4.19 CT of the abdomen showing marked thickening and submucosal oedema of the colon (arrow). Note pneumatosis (arrowhead) within one segment of the bowel wall.

Treatment
Systemic anticoagulation, angioplasty or stenting may be employed. In advanced cases surgical excision of the infarcted segment is required.

4.10 Inflammatory bowel disease – Crohn's disease

Crohn's disease (CD) is a chronic inflammatory disease of the GI tract, characterised by ulceration, strictures and fistula formation. CD commonly affects young adults and typically runs a chronic relapsing–remitting course. Presenting features include diarrhoea, weight loss, malabsorption, anal tags, fistulae and fissures. CD affects 1 in 1200 people in the UK.

Key facts
- CD can affect any part of the GI tract from the mouth to the anal canal, although most cases involve the ileocaecal region (95%)
- The presence of clearly defined normal intestinal segments between diseased segments (termed 'skip lesions') is considered pathognomonic of CD.

Radiological findings

Barium examination The classic finding in CD is that of segmental areas of ileocolic ulceration and thickening. Ulceration ranges from aphthous ulcers in the early stage to deep fissuring transmural ulcers in the advanced stages (**Figure 4.20**).

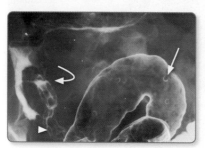

Figure 4.20 Barium enema examination showing aphthous ulcers (arrow), polypoid lesions forming a cobblestone pattern (arrowhead) and stricture in the terminal ileum (curved arrow), which is known as the string sign.

Aphthous ulcers are seen as 'target' or 'bull's-eye'-type lesions, transmural ulcers are seen as penetrating tracks of barium within the bowel wall, and confluent ulcers create a cobblestone pattern of the mucosa.

In the chronic phase strictures may form due to intestinal fibrosis. Luminal narrowing due to inflammation and strictures is termed the 'string sign' and is commonly seen in the ileocaecal region (**Figure 4.21**). Fistulae are seen connecting separate loops of bowel or opening out on to the skin surface.

CT/MRI Fistulae, sinuses and abscesses are better delineated with CT or MRI (**Figure 4.22**). Engorged mesenteric vessels supplying the inflamed bowel segment form the 'comb sign'.

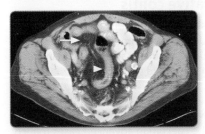

Figure 4.21 CT image of the abdomen shows thickened ileum (arrowhead). Note linearly arranged, engorged blood vessels forming the comb sign (arrow).

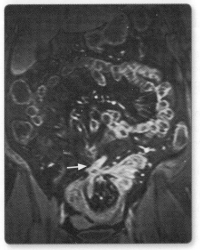

Figure 4.22 Coronal MR scan of the abdomen showing interloop fistula (arrow).

Key imaging findings

A. Aphthous ulcers
B. Fissuring ulcers
C. Cobble-stone mucosa
D. Comb sign

Treatment

Medical treatment is with anti-inflammatory or biological agents. Surgical excision is used in non-refractory CD or obstruction due to strictures.

4.11 Inflammatory bowel disease – ulcerative colitis

Ulcerative colitis (UC) is a diffuse, chronic inflammatory disorder of the colon mucosa. UC is more common than CD and affects 1 in 500 people in the UK. Diarrhoea, malaise, pyrexia and rectal bleeding are common presenting symptoms.

Key facts

- UC typically involves the rectosigmoid with extension proximally up to the caecum in advanced cases (pancolitis)
- One third of patients may have non-specific terminal ileitis (termed 'backwash ileitis') because inflammation refluxes from caecum to the ileum
- The risk of developing colorectal cancer is up to 20 times greater in patients with UC than in the normal population
- Other diseases associated with UC include sclerosing cholangitis, cholangiocarcinoma, ankylosing spondylitis, uveitis and pyoderma gangrenosum.

Radiological findings

Barium examination Mucosal ulcerations cause a granular appearance, and small collar-button ulcers are present (**Figure 4.23**). There is loss of definition of the haustral folds. Polypoid changes are also present due to islands of normal mucosa in between ulcerated areas (pseudopolyps) or true inflammatory polyps. In the chronic stage strictures are present. Haustrations may be lost leading to a 'lead-pipe' colon appearance (**Figure 4.24**).

CT On CT or MRI there is concentric thickening of the colonic wall. In the acute phase there is oedema of the surrounding pericolic fat and increased contrast enhancement due to inflammatory hyperaemia.

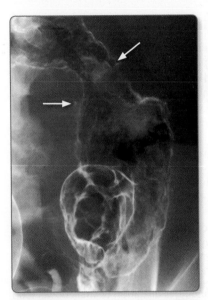

Figure 4.23 Barium enema examination showing small collar-button-type penetrating ulcers (arrows) in the ascending colon.

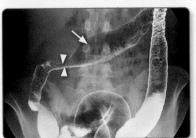

Figure 4.24 Barium enema examination showing loss of haustrations and granular mucosa (arrow). This appearance is termed the 'lead-pipe colon'. Stricture is also present (arrowheads).

Key imaging findings
A. Granular mucosa
B. Collar-button ulcers
C. Strictures
D. Lead-pipe colon

Treatment

Treatment is via medical therapy or surgical colectomy.

4.12 Obstruction – small bowel

Small bowel obstruction (SBO) accounts for up to 80% of cases of intestinal obstruction. Adhesions are the most common cause of SBO followed by hernias. Presentation is typically with intense colicky pain, abdominal distension with high-pitched intestinal sounds and vomiting.

Key facts

- Intestinal adhesions are the causative factor in up to 80% of cases of SBO
- Other causes include hernias (commonly inguinal and femoral), gallstone ileus and secondary tumour involvement (metastases)
- One third of cases due to hernias may be complicated with ischaemia or strangulation.

Radiological findings

Radiograph Classic finding is dilatation of small bowel loop to >3 cm (**Figure 4.25**). Multiple fluid levels (more than three) are present (**Figure 4.26**). The 'string of beads' sign may be seen produced by small pockets of air within an obstructed, fluid-filled, bowel segment. Dilated loops are seen centrally within the abdomen.

CT CT demonstrates dilated bowel loops with abrupt cut-off or change in calibre at the level of the obstruction in cases with adhesions (**Figure 4.27**). CT can also show the 'small-bowel faeces' sign, which is defined by the presence of particulate

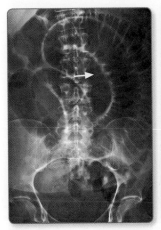

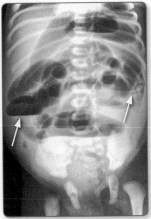

Figure 4.25 Radiograph showing dilated, centrally located bowel loops (arrow) with valvulae conniventes, consistent with small bowel obstruction.

Figure 4.26 Radiograph showing multiple fluid levels (arrows) secondary to bowel obstruction.

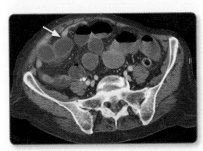

Figure 4.27 CT scan showing abrupt transition from dilated to collapsed (arrow) loops in a case with small bowel obstruction with adhesions. Note multiple fluid levels in the dilated small bowel.

(stool-like) matter within the small bowel. This is due to delayed transit and incompletely digested food, bacterial overgrowth or increased water absorption in the obstructed segment (**Figure 4.28**). Gallstones, hernias and tumours causing SBO are readily demonstrated – gallstones as hyperdense, rounded opacities at the site of blockage with pneumobilia (gas in the bile ducts) (**Figure 4.29**). External hernias are seen as bowel in

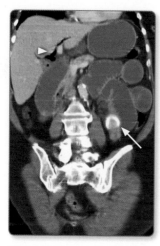

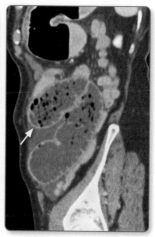

Figure 4.28 CT scan showing small bowel obstruction secondary to gallstone (arrow). Note air within the bile ducts (arrowhead).

Figure 4.29 CT scan showing faeces-like material in a dilated small bowel loop (small bowel faeces sign) (arrow).

the inguinal canal or adjacent to femoral vessels. Ischaemic or strangulated bowel demonstrates lack of normal contrast enhancement on CT.

Key imaging findings

A. Bowel dilatation >3 cm
B. Multiple fluid levels (more than three)
C. Abrupt change in calibre of bowel
D. Small bowel faeces sign.

Treatment

This is nasogastric tube placement with suction. In some cases, especially with perforation, surgical exploration is needed.

4.13 Obstruction – large bowel

Large bowel obstruction (LBO) may present as an emergency that requires early and accurate diagnosis. High-grade colonic obstruction can cause perforation with faecal peritonitis, which can result in high morbidity and mortality. Presentation is with abdominal distension and pain, with the pain possibly being infraumbilical in LBO. Diarrhoea (overflow or due to partial obstruction) may be present and vomiting is not usually a feature.

> ### Clinical insight
>
> CT remains the gold standard in the diagnosis of location and causative factor of SBO and LBO, and is also invaluable in monitoring for complications such as strangulation and ischaemic changes with high accuracy.

Key facts

- The most common aetiological factor causing large bowel obstruction is colorectal cancer
- Other common factors include diverticular disease, volvulus, inflammatory bowel disease and bowel ischaemia.

Radiological findings

Radiograph The colon is distended and usually measures >5 cm (**Figure 4.30**). If it exceeds 9 cm it is termed a 'toxic megacolon' and implies impending perforation. Distended bowel is seen in both flanks, with haustral markings, whereas SBO appears as centrally dilated loops with no haustral markings (**Table 4.1**).

CT On CT the colon appears dilated proximal to the obstruction (**Figure 4.31**). In patients with a competent ileocaecal valve, there may be marked distension of the caecum due to accumulated back pressure from the obstructive site.

Small bowel obstruction	Large bowel obstruction
Central dilated loops	Peripheral dilated loops
Valvulae conniventes	Haustrations
> 3 cm	> 5 cm
String of beads sign	
Small bowel faeces sign	

Table 4.1 Small bowel versus large bowel obstruction

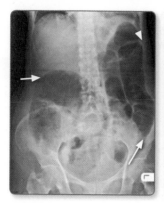 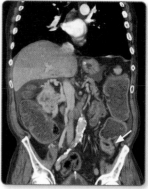

Figure 4.30 Radiograph showing large bowel obstruction with dilated bowel loops (short arrow) located peripherally (long arrow) and with haustral markings (arrowhead).

Figure 4.31 Coronal CT scan showing colon cancer (arrow) causing proximal colonic obstruction.

Key imaging findings

A. Bowel dilatation >5 cm
B. Presence of haustral markings
C. Location along periphery or flanks
D. Toxic megacolon usually >9 cm.

Treatment

Surgical exploration or decompression.

4.14 Oesophageal cancer

Oesophageal cancers are mainly of two types: squamous cell carcinomas (SCCs) or adenocarcinomas. Presenting symptoms may include dysphagia, odynophagia, retrosternal pain, anorexia, anaemia and weight loss.

Key facts

- Approximately two thirds are SCCs and frequently occur in the middle third of the oesophagus

- One third are adenocarcinomas and occur in the distal oesophagus and the gastro-oesophageal junction
- Smoking, alcohol, coeliac disease, GERD and head and neck cancers are all predisposing factors.

Radiological findings

Barium examination Early or small cancers are seen as sessile polyps of plaques. Lack of normal peristalsis and distensibility of the affected segment are also associated with malignant lesions. Advanced lesions show irregular narrowing of the lumen, causing a stricture to form ('rat-tail' strictures) (**Figure 4.32**). Advanced lesions may also have a complex polypoid appearance with ulceration.

CT CT is useful for looking for local spread and invasion of adjacent mediastinal structures (**Figure 4.33**). The normal oesophageal wall measures <3 mm. PET-CT is routinely used to

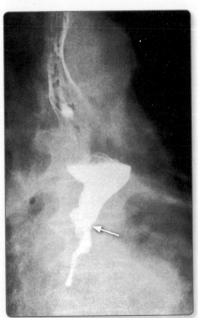

Figure 4.32 Barium swallow examination showing an irregular stricture (arrow) of the lower oesophagus due to cancer.

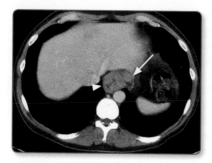

Figure 4.33 CT image shows circumferential thickening of the oesophagus (arrowhead). Enlarged lymph node is seen adjacent to the tumour (arrow).

evaluate lymphatic involvement. Endoscopic US may be used to evaluate local spread more accurately if needed.

Key imaging findings
A. Sessile polyp or plaques
B. Rat-tail stricture
C. Large polypoid lesions
D. Thickening of the oesophageal wall >3 mm on CT.

Treatment
Surgical resection combined with/without radiotherapy or chemotherapy. In palliative cases radiological placement of oesophageal stents is performed to alleviate symptoms of dysphagia.

4.15 Oesophageal perforation (Boerhaave's syndrome)

Oesophageal rupture due to vomiting is termed 'Boerhaave's syndrome'. It is rapidly fatal if not treated promptly and the mortality rate in untreated patients reaches up to 70%. Presentation is with severe chest pain, vomiting and subcutaneous emphysema of the chest and neck.

Key facts
- Boerhaave's syndrome occurs due to sudden massive increase in intraluminal pressure, typically after an alcoholic binge and retching/vomiting

- The rupture is typically located in the distal oesophagus along the left side because this is the weakest, unsupported part of the oesophagus
- Boerhaave's syndrome accounts for 10–15% of oesophageal perforations, the most common factor being iatrogenic perforation (55%).

Radiological findings

Chest radiograph   The key finding is pneumomediastinum (air within the mediastinum), seen as streaks of air outlining the aortic arch or descending aorta, sometimes with associated mediastinal widening. The classic sign associated with perforation is Naclerio V sign, a V-shaped lucency due to air outlining the medial left hemidiaphragm and descending aorta (**Figure 4.34**). Left-sided pleural effusions are also common.

Water-soluble contrast swallow   Contrast extravasates from the oesophagus into the mediastinal and pleural spaces (**Figure 4.35**).

Key imaging findings

A. Pneumomediastinum
B. Naclerio V sign
C. Mediastinal widening and left-sided effusion
D. Leakage of contrast on swallow examination.

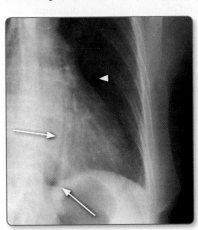

Figure 4.34 Chest radiograph showing pneumomediastinum adjacent to the left heart border (arrowhead). There is a V-shaped lucency along the aorta and diaphragm (arrows).

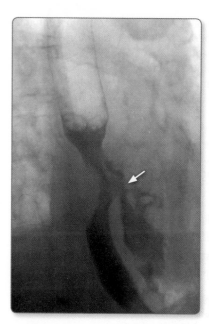

Figure 4.35 Contrast swallow examinations showing leak of contrast from oesophageal perforation (arrow).

Treatment

Small perforations may heal spontaneously. Large perforations need surgical closure and mediastinal/pleural drainage.

4.16 Oesophageal varices

Varices represent dilated subepithelial veins of the oesophagus. In most cases this condition is caused by portal hypertension – usually due to cirrhosis – and the increased blood flow causes dilatation of these veins. Varices are asymptomatic but up to 30% may present with upper GI bleeding that requires emergency treatment.

Key facts

- In patients with liver disease and portal hypertension, varices are seen in the lower two thirds of the oesophagus

- In cases with superior vena cava obstruction, varices are seen in the upper third.

Radiological findings

Barium examination Varices may be seen best on double-contrast barium examinations. They appear as thickened, nodular, longitudinal folds in the oesophagus, with larger ones having a beaded appearance. Extensive varices may create a 'worm-eaten' appearance of the oesophagus (**Figure 4.36**).

CT Larger varices may also be detected on CT as serpiginous, enhancing vessels around the oesophagus.

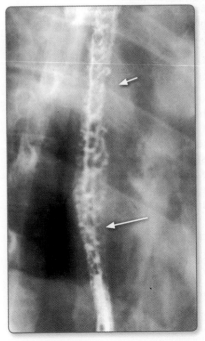

Figure 4.36 Barium swallow shows multiple tortuous filling defects in the oesophagus (arrows) due to varices. The entire oesophagus has a worm-eaten appearance.

Key imaging findings

A. Thickened folds in the oesophagus
B. Beaded or serpiginous folds
C. 'Worm-eaten' appearance
D. Enhancing vessels around
the oesophagus on CT.

Clinical insight

Varices become more prominent during Valsalva's manoeuvre and this procedure may be performed during barium examinations to demonstrate varices.

Treatment

Endoscopic banding or sclerotherapy of bleeding varices.

4.17 Peptic ulceration

Peptic ulcers are one of the most common GI disorders, and it is estimated that 25% of all individuals develop ulcers during their lifetime, although only a small proportion seek medical treatment. Presentation may be with abdominal pain, dyspepsia and heartburn.

Key facts

- Ulcers are most common in middle-aged/elderly individuals, people with alcohol problems and those who use analgesics
- Most ulcers are associated with *H. pylori* and are most common in the distal stomach along the lesser curvature and the first part of the duodenum
- Duodenal ulcers are invariably benign whereas gastric ulcers may be benign or malignant (**Table 4.2**)

Benign gastric ulcer	Malignant gastric ulcer
Barium protrudes beyond the stomach outline	Does not protrude
No adjacent nodules or masses	Sits on a mass
Round or oval	Irregular contour

Table 4.2 Benign versus malignant ulcers.

Radiological findings

Barium examination (Figures 4.37 and **4.38)** Most are round/
elliptical in appearance and are seen as small collections of
barium within the ulcer crater (**Figure 4.37**). Converging folds

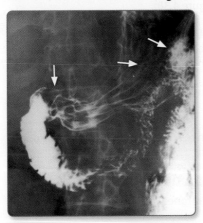

Figure 4.37 Barium
examination showing
round, target-shaped
ulcers in the stomach
(arrows).

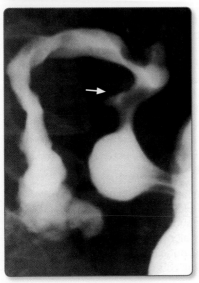

Figure 4.38 Barium
examination showing
scarring of the duodenum
after an ulcer, creating
a trifoliate appearance
(arrow).

may be seen due to collagenous tissue in the base of the ulcer. Oedema around the ulcer may create an ulcer mound. Duodenal ulcers may cause scarring and deformity of the duodenal cap, which may cause a triangular or trifoliate appearance of the duodenal cap (**Figure 4.38**).

Key imaging findings

A. Crater containing barium
B. Round or oval shape
C. Ulcer mound
D. Trifoliate appearance of duodenal cap.

Treatment

Treatment is based on relief of symptoms using antacids and eradication of *H. pylori*.

4.18 Perforation of the GI tract

Free air within the peritoneal cavity (pneumoperitoneum).

Key facts

- Pneumoperitoneum almost always implies perforation of the GI tract, the most common cause of which is a perforated peptic ulcer
- Other aetiological factors include perforation secondary to bowel obstruction and diverticular perforation.

Radiological findings

Chest radiograph The most common finding on erect radiographs is that of free air under the diaphragm (**Figure 4.39**). Very small amounts of free air (<5 ml) can be detected on the erect chest radiograph.

Radiograph On supine views several other signs may be elicited. Air outlining both sides of the bowel wall is termed 'Rigler's sign' (**Figure 4.40**). Air outlining the liver's falciform ligament forms a linear opacity along the right paravertebral region (**Figure 4.41**), whereas outlining of the umbilical ligaments forms an 'inverted V sign'. Lots of air may form a 'football sign',

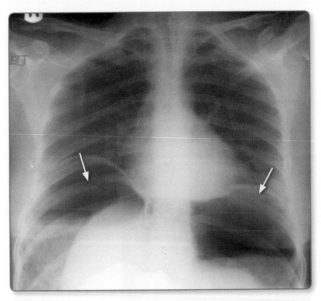

Figure 4.39 Chest radiograph showing free air under both diaphragms (arrows) in a case with pneumoperitoneum.

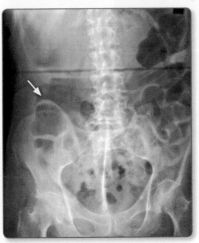

Figure 4.40 Radiograph showing air outlining the outside of the colonic wall forming Rigler's sign (arrow).

which is due to a large ovoid collection of air anteriorly in the abdomen (**Figure 4.42**). Air within mesenteric leaves forms triangular lucent areas. Other common findings may include

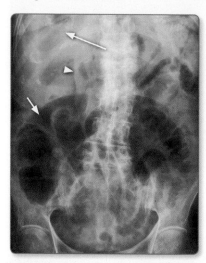

Figure 4.41 Radiograph showing air outlining the falciform ligament (arrowhead) and gas over the liver surface (long arrow). Note how air creates triangular shadows between the mesenteric leaves and bowel (short arrow).

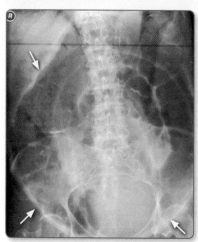

Figure 4.42 Radiograph showing the 'football sign' (arrows) due to large amount of air in the peritoneum.

collections of air over the liver shadow.

CT In equivocal cases CT provides confirmatory information.

Key imaging findings

A. Free air under diaphragm
B. Rigler's sign
C. Outlining of ligaments
D. Air over liver surface

Treatment

Treatment is based on the cause of the pneumoperitoneum.

Clinical scenario

- An 86-year-old woman presented on New Year's Day with sudden onset of right lower quadrant pain, abdominal distension and vomiting. She had had low-grade pain in her abdomen since Christmas, which was getting worse. The radiograph was unhelpful. A CT showed thickened loops of bowel in the right lower quadrant. A linear density is seen within one of the bowel loops (**Figure 4.43**).

- This was a piece of turkey bone. Swallowed foreign bodies such as fish bones or chicken bones can cause obstruction and bowel perforation. Bones may be swallowed by elderly, edentulous patients.

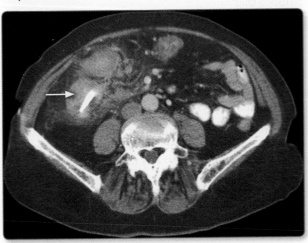

Figure 4.43 CT scan showing thickened bowel loops with a linear hyperdensity (arrow).

4.19 Pseudomembranous colitis

Pseudomembranous colitis (PMC) is also known as antibiotic-associated diarrhoea. In this condition, multiple, elevated, yellowish plaques are seen on the colonic mucosa which are called pseudomembranes. Patients typically have a history of recent antibiotic use and present with diarrhoea and lower abdominal pain. PMC may occur even after a single dose of antibiotics or even 3–4 months after exposure to antibiotics.

Key facts

- Antibiotic therapy is the key factor that alters the colonic flora allowing *Clostridium difficile (C. dif)* to flourish
- Acquired nosocomial infection is particularly common in hospitals and nursing homes
- Toxins produced by the gut pathogen *C. dif* cause PMC
- Pseudomembranes are formed due to sloughed off mucosa and exudates composed of inflammatory debris and white blood cells.

Radiological findings

Radiograph The main radiological finding is marked thickening of the colonic wall with nodularity of haustra. Contiguous involvement of the entire colon may be seen starting from the rectosigmoid up to the caecum. Isolated involvement of colonic segments is rare.

CT CT has high positive predictive value in the detection of PMC (90%) and is the imaging modality of choice. The classic appearance is that of a markedly thickened colonic wall with contrast trapped between the colonic folds, forming the 'accordion' sign (**Figure 4.44**). The marked thickening is due to excessive submucosal oedema in the colonic wall. The colon may be markedly dilated (toxic megacolon) in severe cases and may perforate. Ascites is commonly present and may be seen in up to 35–40% of patients, whereas it is uncommon in other inflammatory conditions of the colon.

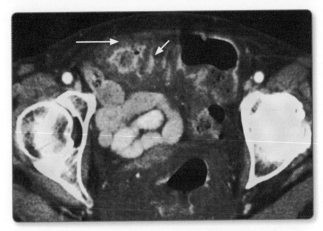

Figure 4.44 CT image shows marked thickening of the colon (long arrow) due to submucosal oedema. Oral contrast trapped within thickened haustra creates the accordion sign (short arrow)

Key imaging findings

A. Marked thickening and nodularity of the colonic wall and haustra
B. Accordion sign on CT
C. Toxic megacolon in severe cases
D. Ascites commonly seen

Treatment

In mild cases, withdrawal of the offending antibiotic can suffice. In severe cases metronidazole or vancomycin therapy may be required.

4.20 Scleroderma

Scleroderma (progressive systemic sclerosis) is a multisystem autoimmune disorder involving the skin, synovium and parenchyma of multiple organs. GI tract changes are the third most common manifestation of this disease, after skin changes and Raynaud's phenomenon (episodic vasospasmic blanching, pain and cyanosis of the digits when exposed to the cold). Symptoms may include dysphagia, epigastric fullness, abdominal pain and bloating.

Key facts

- GI tract involvement (mainly oesophagus and small bowel) is seen in up to 90% of patients and is a common cause of chronic intestinal pseudo-obstruction (decreased ability of the intestine to push food through due to abnormalities in muscle tone and peristalsis)
- Scleroderma can be associated with other conditions such as systemic lupus erythematosus, dermatomyositis and CREST syndrome (calcinosis, Raynaud's phenomenon, oesophageal dysmotility, sclerodactyly and telangiectasia).

Radiological findings

Barium examination Normal peristalsis is observed in the upper third of the oesophagus whereas the lower two thirds is atonic or aperistaltic. The oesophagus is dilated and may have ulcers at its lower end due to acid reflux caused by a gastro-oesophageal junction that is open widely.

There is marked dilatation of the small bowel, particularly the duodenum and proximal jejunum (**Figure 4.45**), which along with crowded, stretched mucosal folds give a pathognomonic 'hide-bound' appearance. This occurs due to muscular atrophy and its replacement by collagen in the submucosal layer of the bowel. Multiple diverticula may be seen arising from the small bowel, and there is also marked delay in transit of barium through the bowel.

Key imaging findings

A. Dilated oesophagus
B. Wide open LES
C. Lower oesophageal ulcers from reflux
D. 'Hide-bound appearance'

Treatment

This is antacid treatment for reflux disease. Medical treatment to promote normal gut motility.

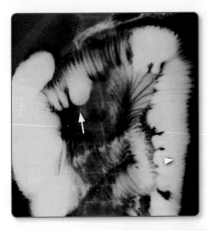

Figure 4.45 Barium examination showing marked dilatation of the duodenum (arrow) and proximal jejunum with stretched mucosal folds (arrowhead), creating the hide-bound sign.

4.21 Tuberculosis of the GI tract

GI tract tuberculosis (TB) is caused by ingestion of infected sputum, via haematological or local spread. Patient may present with pain, weight loss, fever, palpable masses and ascites.

Key facts

TB can affect any part of the bowel but the ileocaecal junction is the most commonly affected site, due to the abundance of lymphoid tissue (Peyer's patches) in the distal and terminal ileum.

Radiological findings

Barium examination In the small bowel, nodular, thickened and distorted folds around the ileocaecal junction can be seen. As with Crohn's disease, deep fissures, sinus tracts, enterocutaneous fistulae and perforation can less commonly occur. Ulceration may be demonstrated, typically along the circumference of the bowel wall. Caecum is often involved more severely than the terminal ileum (**Figure 4.46**). Chronic disease can show caecal contraction with loss of normal angle at the ileocaecal junction and a patulous ileocaecal valve. The ileum empties into a deformed cone-shaped caecum at right angles with hypertrophy of the ileocecal valve (Fleischner's sign) (**Figure 4.47**). Colonic involvement causes deep ulceration

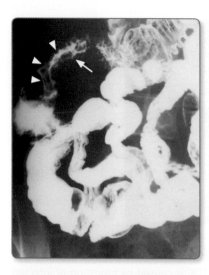

Figure 4.46 Barium examination shows irregularity of the ileocaecal region (arrowheads) with oval ulcers (arrow).

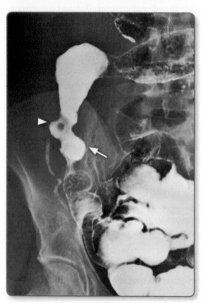

Figure 4.47 Barium examination shows a contracted caecum (arrowhead) which has retracted upwards with loss of normal acute angle of the ileocaecal junction (arrow).

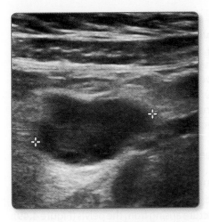

Figure 4.48 US scan of the right iliac fossa howing a necrotic node in the same patient as Figure 4.47.

and mucosal granulation, leading to nodularity, inflammatory polyps and hour-glass-shaped strictures.

US/CT TB is almost invariably associated with caseating and necrotic lymphadenopathy and peritoneal inflammation with ascites (**Figure 4.48**).

Key imaging findings
A. Thickened folds and ulcers
B. Ileocaecal involvement
C. Fleischner's sign
D. Strictures in small and large bowel

Treatment
Treatment of GI tract TB is with anti-tubercular drug treatment.

4.22 Volvulus of the colon

Volvulus of the colon occurs due to twisting of the bowel around itself. This is most common in the sigmoid colon and is the third most common cause of LBO in many reported series. Patients usually present with abdominal distension, pain and vomiting.

Key facts

- Torsion of the colon usually occurs in the setting of a congenitally long, mobile mesentery
- Other predisposing factors include chronic constipation when patients develop a large, elongated, relatively atonic colon that is prone to twist on itself
- The volvulus is most commonly sited in the sigmoid (60–70%), whereas caecal volvulus is the second most common site (up to 30%)
- Rarely there may be a volvulus of the transverse colon.

Radiological findings

Radiograph Sigmoid volvulus appears as a dilated 'C-' or 'U-shaped' gas-filled structure arising from the pelvis (**Figure 4.49**). The apex of the dilated bowel is commonly located under the left diaphragm, and no haustrations are usually seen. Another useful finding is the 'coffee-bean' sign, referring to the shape of

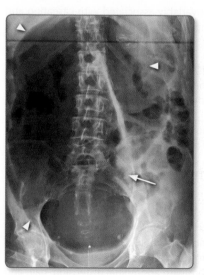

Figure 4.49 Radiograph showing a large, ahaustral, distended bowel loop (arrow) arising from the pelvis. It has a lenticular, coffee-bean shape (arrowheads).

the dilated sigmoid colon. Caecal volvulus is seen as a gas-filled, dilated bowel loop, with its apex pointing upwards, usually in the left upper quadrant (**Figure 4.50**). Haustral markings are visible in a caecal volvulus as opposed to the ahaustral appearance of sigmoid volvulus.

CT The distended bowel is again visualised. The point of torsion is seen on CT as a 'whirl sign' consisting of twisted bowel and mesenteric blood vessels (**Figure 4.51**). The abnormal position of the sigmoid colon or caecum and swirling of the mesentery at the level of the volvulus are visible.

Key imaging findings
A. Dilated, ahaustral bowel loop arising from the pelvis
B. Coffee-bean sign
C. Caecal volvulus showing haustrations and with apex in the left upper quadrant
D. Whirl sign on CT.

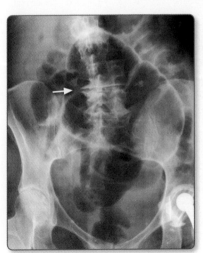

Figure 4.50 Radiograph showing a distended loop with haustral markings, with its apex pointing superiorly (arrow). This is the inverted caecum in a patient with caecal volvulus.

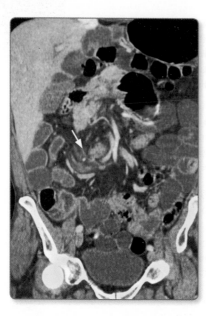

Figure 4.51 Coronal CT scan showing the twisting of vessels (arrow) in a patient with a sigmoid volvulus.

Treatment

In uncomplicated sigmoid volvulus, insertion of a flatus tube per rectum provides adequate decompression. In complicated cases or caecal volvulus surgical correction may be needed.

Genitourinary system 5

The genitourinary system consists of the renal tract and in males includes the reproductive organs such as the prostate, seminal vesicles and testes. The kidneys are responsible for filtering the blood and extracting waste products that are excreted into the urinary bladder via the ureters. Disorders of the kidneys such as cancer may produce haematuria (blood in the urine), whereas poor renal function leads to elevation of serum creatinine and urea levels. Some common diseases affecting the renal tract are urolithiasis (renal stones) and chronic renal failure. In younger patients testicular torsion may present as an emergency. US is commonly the initial imaging modality used in the evaluation of the renal tract. It is also particularly useful for evaluating the scrotal sac. CT plays an important role in diagnosis and staging of renal cancer and renal trauma.

5.1 Renal artery stenosis

Renal artery stenosis (RAS) is the most common cause of secondary hypertension. It is defined as narrowing of the lumen of the renal artery and is most commonly (two thirds) caused by atherosclerotic disease. Fibromuscular dysplasia is the second most common cause of RAS. Patients usually present with very high blood pressure or acute onset of hypertension. A vascular bruit (turbulent flow noise) may be felt or heard in the flanks/abdomen.

Key facts
- Atheromatous plaques and calcification typically occur at the origin or within 2 cm of the origin of the renal artery from the aorta
- Atheromatous RAS affects older men (usually >50 years), and is bilateral in 30% of cases

- Fibromuscular dysplasia is an autosomal dominant disorder affecting younger patients (more often female), causing medial hyperplasia (middle layer) of the arterial wall
- The area of narrowing is usually in the mid or distal renal arteries and is bilateral in two thirds of cases.

Radiological findings

CT or MR angiography Along with traditional catheter angiography, CTA or MRA may be used to delineate the renal vasculature and detect areas of narrowing. Doppler studies can be carried out to assess blood flow velocities through the renal arteries (see Figure 1.19).

Angiography (CT, MR or catheter) Atheromatous stenosis is usually seen as eccentric areas of narrowing at or near the origin of the renal arteries (Figure 5.1). In patients with fibromuscular dysplasia, multiple narrowings are in the mid to distal renal arteries forming a 'string of beads' appearance (Figure 5.2).

US with doppler There is an increase in the systolic peak velocity of blood flow through the renal arteries. A peak velocity >200 cm/s signifies severe (50–99%) occlusion whereas velocities between 100 and 200 cm/s are consistent with modest stenosis (<50%).

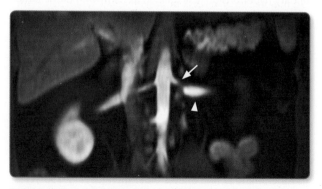

Figure 5.1 MR angiography scan showing stenosis of the left renal artery (arrow) and post-stenotic dilatation (arrowhead).

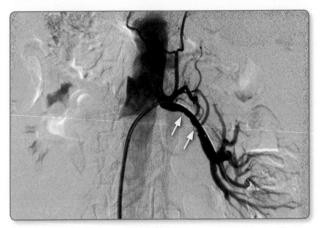

Figure 5.2 Angiographic image showing multiple stenoses (arrows) in the left renal artery forming the string of beads appearance.

Key imaging findings

A. Narrrowing of renal artery
B. Multiple narrowing in fibromuscular dysplasia
C. String of beads appearance
D. Increased flow velocity on Doppler studies (>100 cm/s)

Treatment

RAS may be dilated by balloon angioplasty (PTRA or percutaneous transluminal renal angioplasty). Surgical revascularisation has the best success rate in treating renal artery stenosis.

5.2 Renal cell carcinoma

Renal cell carcinoma (RCC) arises from the tubular epithelium of the kidney and is also known as hypernephroma. It is the most common primary renal tumour (85%) and quite often detected incidentally on CT or US. Symptoms typically include haematuria, flank pain or palpable masses.

Key facts

- RCC is associated with congenital conditions such as von Hippel–Lindau syndrome and tuberous sclerosis

- Distant metastases may be the first presenting sign of RCC and the classic triad of haematuria, flank pain and mass is present in <10% of patients.

Radiological findings

Radiographs A focal bulge on the renal shadow or calcification may be seen on radiographs (**Figure 5.3**).

US RCCs can be hypoechoic or hyperechoic because they may contain cystic areas, septations and solid elements (**Figure 5.4**). High blood flow velocities are seen on Doppler studies due to AV (arteriovenous) shunting within the tumour. Abnormal AV connections and shunts are formed due to neovascularity and angiogenesis in renal tumours.

CT The typical appearance of RCC is that of a hyperenhancing mass located in the renal cortex (**Figure 5.5**). Calcification may be present in up to a third of cases. These tumours are best seen on early arterial phase imaging. Metastases are seen in

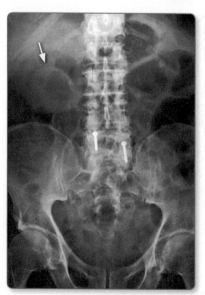

Figure 5.3 Radiograph showing a faintly calcified rounded lesion (arrow) over the right renal shadow.

the lungs or bones. Less common sites are the adrenal glands and the contralateral kidney. CT is also useful for detecting tumour extension into the perinephric fat and tumour-related thrombosis of the renal veins or inferior vena cava (IVC).

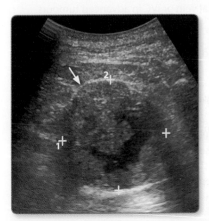

Figure 5.4 US scan showing a solid mass with central necrotic areas (arrow).

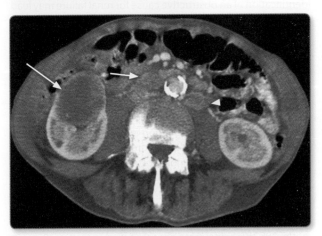

Figure 5.5 Axial CT scan showing a cortically based tumour arising from the right kidney (long arrow). The IVC shows a lack of enhancement suggestive of thrombosis (short arrow). Note metastatic involvement of the left adrenal (arrowhead).

Key imaging findings
A. Focal bulge in renal contour with calcification
B. Renal mass with central necrotic areas on US
C. Cortical-based enhancing mass on CT
D. Thrombosis of renal vein or IVC in advanced tumours.

Treatment

RCCs are best treated by surgical excision including partial nephrectomy.

5.3 Renal failure

Renal failure may be acute (ARF) or chronic (CRF). Imaging in patients with renal failure has two roles:
1. To identify any obstructive lesion
2. To evaluate renal size and cortical thickness because CRF leads to small, atrophic kidneys

Key facts

Identification of an obstructive cause for renal failure may lead to surgical correction, whereas chronic renal failure is usually not correctable.

Radiological findings

US Acute obstruction leads to dilatation of the renal collecting system (hydronephrosis) (**Figure 5.6**). Dilated calyces are seen on US as branching, fluid structures within the renal parenchyma. If an obstructing lesion is not seen on US, CT may provide better assessment of the ureters and bladder.

In cases with ARF and non-obstructed kidney, other diagnoses such as acute tubular necrosis, acute glomerulonephritis or pyelonephritis should be considered. In pyelonephritis the kidney is increased in size and there is poor differentiation of the corticomedullary junctions.

In CRF the kidneys are shrunken and measure <9 cm in length. Normal renal cortex should be less echogenic than the liver, whereas in CRF the cortex becomes increasingly echogenic and may be brighter than the adjacent liver (**Figure 5.7**).

Key imaging findings

A. Hydronephrosis
B. Enlarged kidney in pyelonephritis
C. Shrunken kidney in CRF
D. Echogenic cortex more than in liver in CRF

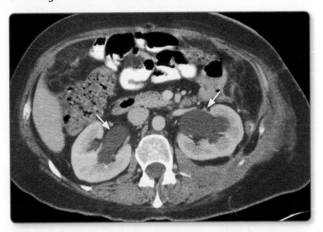

Figure 5.6 CT scans showing bilateral hydronephross (arrows) seen in a patent with acute renal failure.

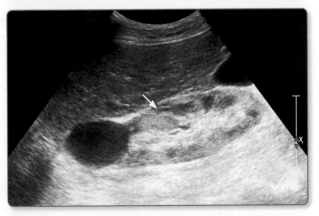

Figure 5.7 US scan showing increased echogenicity of the renal cortex (arrow), as compared with the adjacent liver, in chronic renal failure.

Treatment

Treatment in obstructive ARF is by removal of the offending cause. CRF may need dialysis or transplantation in the long term.

5.4 Trauma – renal injuries

Renal injury usually occurs due to blunt trauma rather than penetrating injury, with kidneys injured in up to 10% of patients with significant abdominal blunt trauma. Clinical presentation may be with flank pain, bruising, haematuria or shock.

Key facts

Kidneys are particularly susceptible to injury in children, because they are not as well protected by the ribs and muscles of the back.

Radiological findings

Renal injuries are graded into four subtypes based on imaging findings (**Figure 5.8a**):

1. Type I injuries (75–85%) involve laceration of the corticomedullary region that does not communicate with the collecting system. On US these appear as hypoechoic, cystic collections. On CT lacerations are hyperdense in the acute phase due to fresh blood but gradually decrease in density (**Figure 5.8b**)
2. Type II injuries (10–15%) are lacerations that communicate with the collecting system. These patients have haematuria and flank masses due to perinephric haematomas. CT demonstrates leakage of contrast medium into perinephric spaces
3. Type III injuries (5%) are major injuries with damage to the vascular pedicle and shattered kidneys. These patients may be too unstable for imaging; however, if needed angiography can demonstrate damage to the renal artery or vein and CT may show non-enhancement of the kidney. Enhancement of the cortical rim is termed the 'subcapsular rim sign' and is seen in complete renal artery occlusion (**Figure 5.9**)
4. Type IV injuries cause injury and avulsion of the pelviureteric junction (**Figure 5.10**). In these cases there is massive extravasation of contrast from the ruptured renal pelvis or ureter.

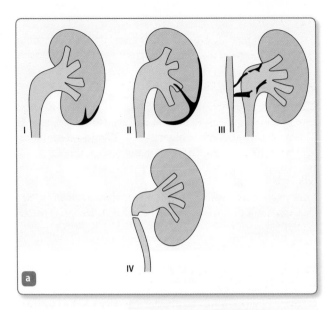

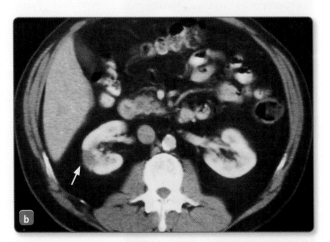

Figure 5.8 (a) The four different types of renal injury. (b) CT scan showing renal contusion as a focal area of non-enhancement in the right kidney (arrow).

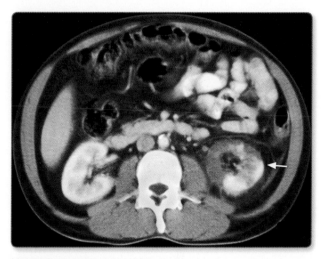

Figure 5.9 CT scans showing lack of enhancement of the left kidney with only peripheral or rim enhancement (arrow).

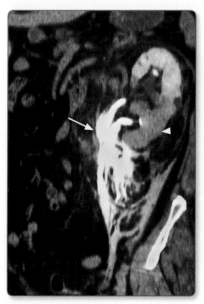

Figure 5.10 CT scan showing pelviureteric disruption with extra-vasation of contrast around the ureters (arrow). Note the complete lack of enhancement of the lower pole of the kidney (arrowhead).

Key imaging findings

A. Hypoechoic or hypodense crescentic or linear areas in the kidney

B. Perinephric haematoma or contrast extravasation

C. Subcapsular rim sign

D. Extravasation from the pelviureteric junction.

Treatment

Type I and II injuries are treated conservatively, except in type II cases in whom there is persistent blood loss or pain. Type III and IV injuries require surgical treatment. Occasionally Type IV injuries may be treated by radiological stent insertion.

5.5 Urolithiasis (renal tract stones)

Most renal stones are composed of calcium and 90% are radio-opaque. Rarely stones are composed of uric acid, xanthine or cystine, and these are usually radiolucent and not detected by X-rays. The typical presentation is with renal colic, i.e. loin-to-groin pain, haematuria and fever. The overall incidence of renal stones in the general population is 12% in males and approximately 4% in females.

Key facts

Most patients presenting with renal colic have ureteric stones and these may be best seen on CT.

Radiological findings

Radiograph Most small calculi may not be visible on radiographs due to overlying structures. Larger calculi are seen as dense opacities projected over the renal shadow or in the ureteric line along the tip of the transverse processes of the spine (**Figures 5.11** and **5.12**).

US This has high sensitivity in detecting renal and bladder calculi. Ureteric stones are difficult to visualise on US due to overlying bowel and other structures. Stones are seen as echogenic structures with posterior acoustic shadowing.

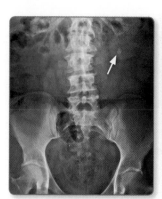

Figure 5.11 Radiograph showing a renal calculus as a dense lesion projected over the left renal shadow (arrow).

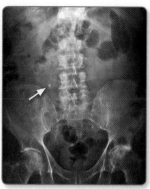

Figure 5.12 Radiograph showing a ureteric calculus along the line of the tip of the transverse process (arrow).

CT The most sensitive examination is non-contrast-enhanced CT of the renal tract. Calculi appear as hyperdense foci within the kidney or ureters, with the 'rim sign' seen with ureteric stones due to oedema around an impacted stone (**Figure 5.13**). Usually there is dilatation of the proximal collecting system (hydronephrosis) and the ureter may also be dilated >5 mm. Contrast may be administered to detect lucent stones (not opaque to X-rays) if needed. Lucent stones are seen as filling defects outlined by contrast in the obstructed segment.

Key imaging findings
A. Hydronephrosis
B. Echogenic stones with posterior shadowing
C. Hyperdense stones on CT
D. Rim sign

Treatment
Treatment is with hydration and extracorporeal shock wave lithotripsy (ESWL). In cases with secondary infection with obstruction, US-guided percutaneous drainage of the kidney may be performed (nephrostomy).

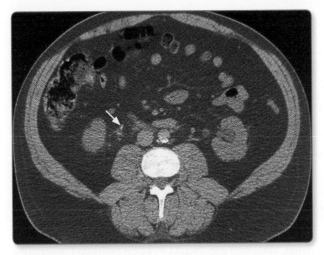

Figure 5.13 CT image showing a dense ureteric stone (arrow) with surrounding soft tissue cuff of oedema forming the 'rim sign'.

5.6 Testicular cancer

Testicular cancer is the most common cancer affecting younger men in the second or third decade of life. The majority are germ-cell tumours and have a high cure rate. Presentation is usually with a painless swelling or lump in the testes. Pain may be present in a minority of patients.

Key facts

1. Most tumours are seminomas followed by teratomas or embryonal cell carcinomas
2. Testicular cancer is associated with cryptorchidism.

Radiological findings

US Cancers are typically seen as hypoechoic lesions within the testes (**Figure 5.14**). Calcification may be seen in teratomatous tumours.

CT CT is used for staging and assessment of lymphadenopathy or distant spread (most often lymph nodes of the

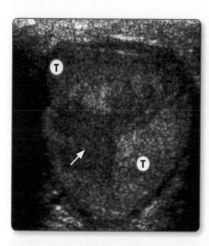

Figure 5.14 US scan showing a testicular cancer as an irregular, hypoechoic lesion (arrow).
Ⓣ testicle.

pelvis, abdomen and thorax). Positron emission tomography (PET)-CT can also be used for follow-up investigations. Any retroperitoneal node >1 cm should be considered abnormal. Non-seminomatous germ-cell tumours (NSGCTs) may cause cystic (hypodense) lymphadenopathy.

Key imaging findings
A. Enlarged testicle
B. Focal hypoechoic lesion
C. Abdominopelvic lymphadenopathy
D. Cystic lymphadenopathy in NSGCT

Treatment
Radical orchidectomy.

5.7 Testicular hydrocoele

This condition is caused by a serous fluid collection between the layers of tunica vaginalis of the scrotum. Hydrocoeles are typically painless swellings that show transillumination.

Key facts
- Hydrocoeles are the most common cause of scrotal enlargement

- When there is a congenital defect in the tunica vaginalis, fluid from the abdomen can collect in the scrotum, causing a communicating hydrocoele
- Acquired hydrocoeles are caused by infections, trauma or torsion
- Up to 10% of testicular tumours are associated with secondary hydrocoeles.

Radiological findings

US The classic appearance of a hydrocoele is an anechoic collection surrounding the testes on US (**Figure 5.15**). The fluid collection may contain septations and scattered echoes caused by protein or cholesterol content (**Figure 5.16**). The areas where rête testis attaches to the epididymis are spared and not surrounded by fluid.

MRI Hydrocoeles are usually composed of serous fluid and show high signal on T2-weighted MRI.

Hydrocoeles may be complicated by secondary infection and then may contain debris and septations. An abnormally large hydrocoele can exert pressure that may compromise

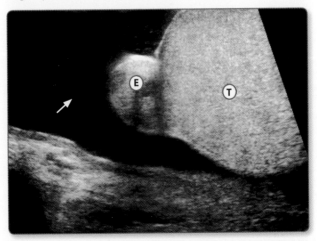

Figure 5.15 US scan showing a hydrocoele as an anechoic fluid collection around the testicle (arrow). (E) epididymis, (T) testicle.

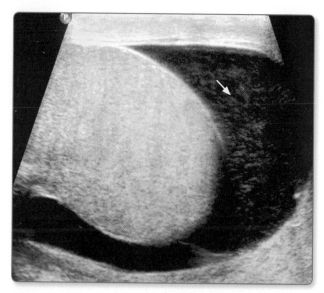

Figure 5.16 US scan showing debris within a hydrocoele as echogenic particles (arrow).

blood flow (lack of blood flow on Doppler studies) within the testis.

Key imaging findings

A. Crescentic anechoic fluid collection
B. Septations and echogenic debris
C. Low signal fluid collection on T1-weighted MRI
D. High signal fluid collection on T2-weighted MRI

Treatment

Surgical excision of the fluid with stitching of the edges of the tunica leads to excellent prognosis.

5.8 Testicular torsion

Testicular torsion is the twisting of the testicle and its spermatic cord leading to ischaemia. Adolescent boys are most often affected and presentation is with acute scrotal pain, tenderness and swelling.

Key facts

- Testicular torsion occurs due to deficient attachment of the testicle to the tunica
- Subsequent torsion of the contralateral testicle is common.

Radiological findings

US US with Doppler imaging is best for diagnosis. The torted testicle is enlarged and has a heterogeneous echotexture (**Figure 5.17**). A hydrocoele is often present, as is decreased or absent blood flow on Doppler scans (**Figure 5.18**). In delayed presentation there may be areas of haemorrhage or necrosis in the testicle, seen as hypoechoic, irregular or cystic areas.

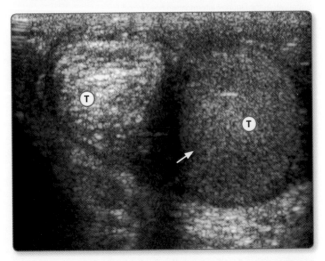

Figure 5.17 US scan showing an enlarged left testicle (arrow) of heterogeneous appearance in a case with torsion. Ⓣ testicle.

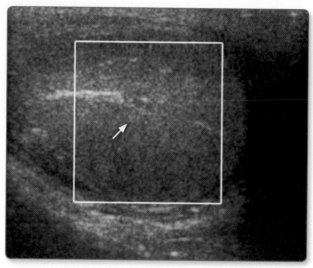

Figure 5.18 Complete loss of blood flow seen as a complete lack of colour signal within the Doppler interrogation box (arrow)

Key imaging findings
A. Enlarged testicle
B. Hydrocoele
C. Absent blood flow
D. Haemorrhage or necrosis

Treatment
Treatment is with surgical intervention and orchidopexy.

5.9 Testicular varicocoele

Testicular varicocoele is formed by dilatation of the pampi-niform plexus of veins around/above the testes. Varicocoeles are an important aetiological factor of low sperm count and therefore male infertility. Usually asymptomatic, presentation may be with infertility or dull ache in the groin.

Key facts

- Up to 10% of men may have varicocoeles, most of which are on the left side
- Uncommon causes include retroperitoneal tumours or renal vein thrombosis causing testicular vein obstruction.

Radiological findings

US Varicocoeles are best investigated by US. They are seen as multiple tortuous structures at the upper pole of the testes (**Figure 5.19**). The dilated veins are >3 mm in diameter and increase in size on Valsalva's manoeuvre. Serpiginous dilated veins may also be seen on other imaging investigations such as CT or MRI.

Key imaging findings

A. Multiple, tubular, serpiginous structures
B. Blood flow on Doppler studies
C. Increase in diameter on Valsalva's manoeuvre
D. Common on the left side

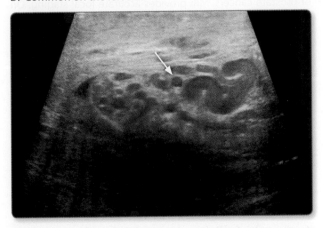

Figure 5.19 US scan showing a varicocoele as multiple, tubular, serpiginous abnormalities (arrow).

Treatment

Treatment is with surgical ligation or transcatheter embolisation.

5.10 Prostatic cancer

Prostate cancer is the most common cancer affecting males and a major cause of death in elderly men. Most tumours are adenocarcinomas and >70% occur in the peripheral zone of the gland. Patients may be asymptomatic or present with urinary symptoms such as hesitancy, frequency or urgency.

Key facts

- Prostate cancer can spread via lymph or blood
- Rounded 'canon-ball' secondaries are seen in the lungs whereas bone lesions are typically sclerotic in appearance.

Radiological findings

US Transrectal US is widely used for diagnosis and biopsy of prostate cancers. MRI provides accurate local staging. On transrectal US tumours have a hypoechoic appearance (**Figure 5.20**). The prostate gland may be enlarged in size or may show asymmetrical contour changes.

MRI On MRI cancers are seen as areas of low signal on T2-weighted sequences against the normal high signal from the normal prostatic tissue (**Figure 5.21**). The strength of MRI lies in detection of extraprostatic spread, which usually starts at the right and left posterolateral zones along the anatomical locations of the neurovascular bundles. Extension is seen as a capsular bulge with irregular margins, contour abnormalities or direct breach of the capsule with tumour spread. Prostatic secondary to bones may be best evaluated using nuclear bone scans (**Figure 5.22**).

Key imaging findings

A. Enlarged prostate
B. Hypoechoic area in the peripheral zone

C. Hypointense on T2-weighted MRI

D. Capsular bulging and breach of capsule

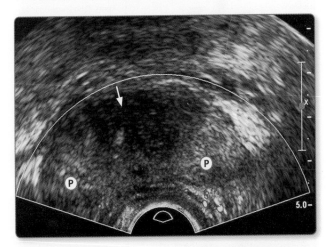

Figure 5.20 Transrectal US scan showing a hypoechoic lesion (arrow) in the prostate Ⓟ consistent with tumour.

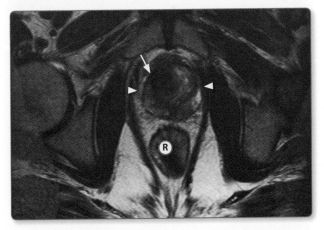

Figure 5.21 MR scan showing hypointense tumour (arrow) within an enlarged prostate (arrowheads). Ⓡ rectum.

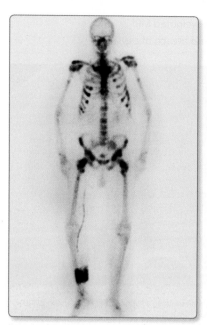

Figure 5.22 Nuclear scan showing multiple skeletal prostatic metastases as hot spots. (The linear opacity along the right leg is the isotope draining out from the bladder into the urinary bag).

Treatment
Hormonal therapy or radical prostatectomy.

5.11 Benign prostatic hyperplasia

Benign prostatic hyperplasia (BPH) is a non-cancerous enlargement of the prostate gland characterised by proliferation of its epithelial and stromal cellular elements. It usually presents with lower urinary tract symptoms such as urinary frequency, urgency, a weak and intermittent stream, and nocturia. BPH may lead to complications such as acute urinary retention.

Key facts

- The development of BPH is considered to be hormonally dependent on testosterone and dihydrotestosterone (DHT) production
- Almost half of all men demonstrate histopathological BPH by the age of 60 years.

Radiological findings

US This is used to determine the prostate size. Transrectal US is recommended in patients with elevated prostate-specific antigen levels along with transrectal biopsy if needed. Intravesicle enlargement of the prostate causes a smooth filling defect to appear within the bladder (**Figure 5.23**). Bladder outlet obstruction leads to thickening and trabeculation of the bladder wall. The prostate appears nodular with hypoechoic or mixed echotexture.

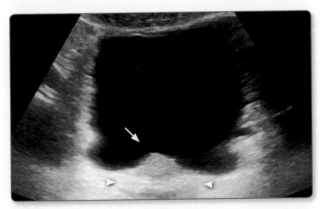

Figure 5.23 US scan showing enlargement of the prostate (arrowheads) with projection of the median lobe into the bladder (arrow).

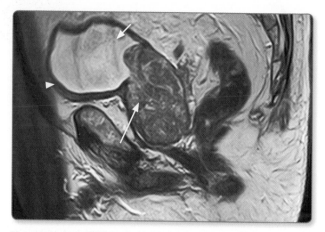

Figure 5.24 Sagittal MRI image shows enlarged prostate (arrow) as a lobulated, cystic organ with projection into the bladder (short arrow). Note thickened bladder wall (arrowhead).

MRI MRI shows an enlarged prostate with high signal intensity and cystic changes (**Figure 5.24**).

Key imaging findings

A. Enlarged prostate
B. Filling defect in the bladder base
C. Thickened and trabeculated bladder
D. Nodular echotexture on transrectal US

Treatment

Treatment may be medical in patients with mild symptoms, including use of α-adrenergic receptor-blocking agents that decrease resistance along the bladder neck, prostate and urethra by relaxing the smooth muscles. Surgical treatment includes transurethral resection of the prostate (TURP).

Hepatobiliary system

The hepatobiliary system consists of the liver, gallbladder, bile ducts, pancreas and spleen. The liver is the largest organ in the abdomen, weighing 1200–1500 g. The gallbladder functions to store and concentrate bile produced by the liver. The pancreas is both an endocrine gland producing hormones such as insulin and an exocrine gland secreting digestive enzymes which help to break down carbohydrates, fat and proteins. The spleen has an important regulatory function in maintaining red blood cells (RBCs); it removes old RBCs, holds a reserve of blood and recycles iron. It also produces antibodies and removes antibody-coated bacteria via the blood and lymphatic circulations. A wide variety of clinical disorders affect the hepatobiliary system, common disorders including biliary and gallbladder stones, hepatitis, cirrhosis and pancreatitis. US is usually the first-line modality for evaluation of hepatobiliary disorders. MRI and CT play a crucial role in characterising lesions and evaluating disorders in greater detail.

6.1 Cholecystitis

Cholecystitis is almost always caused by gallstones obstructing the cystic duct. Only a minority of cases are termed 'acalculous cholecystitis' (<5%). Patients typically present with colicky right upper quadrant (RUQ) pain and leukocytosis.

Key facts

- Pain and tenderness on compression during inhalation in the RUQ are termed 'Murphy's sign'
- This sign may also be elicited on US using the US probe to compress the gallbladder under direct vision – 'sonographic Murphy's sign'
- Cholesterol is the main component in approximately 80% of gallstones.

Radiological findings

Radiograph As gallstones degenerate, nitrogen gas may collect in their central fissures, producing the 'Mercedes-Benz' sign on radiographs. Occasionally calcified, faceted gallstones may be seen.

US US remains the gold standard for gallbladder stones. There is a highly reflective echo from the anterior surface of the gallstone, the stone is mobile on repositioning the patient and there is marked posterior acoustic shadowing (**Figure 6.1**). Even small (<3 mm) asymptomatic stones can be detected with US. If the gallbladder is full of stones, a 'wall–echo–shadow (WES)' sign is demonstrated (**Figure 6.2**). This is formed by the anterior wall of the gallbladder, the highly echogenic surface of gallstones and then the associated posterior shadowing. The gallbladder wall is usually thickened, measuring >4 mm. Pericholecystic fluid may be present (**Figure 6.3**). Stones impacted at the cystic duct may cause extrinsic compression and obstruction of the

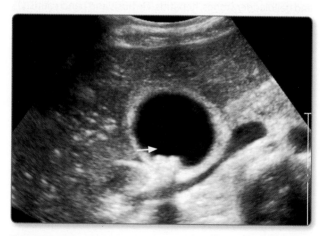

Figure 6.1 US scan showing stones (arrow) within a thickened gallbladder. Note that stones cause posterior acoustic shadowing.

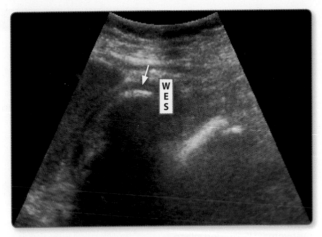

Figure 6.2 The WES sign (arrow) formed by echoes from the gallbladder wall (W), echo from stone (E) and posterior shadow (S).

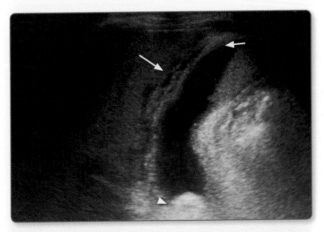

Figure 6.3 US scan showing marked gallbladder thickening (short arrow) with pericholecystic fluid (long arrow). Note calculus (arrowhead) obstructing the neck of the gallbladder.

common bile duct (Mirizzi's syndrome).

Key imaging findings

A. Gallstones
B. WES sign
C. Thickened gallbladder wall
D. Pericholecystic inflammation and fluid

Treatment

Treatment is usually by surgical cholecystectomy. In frail or severely ill patients with empyema, US-guided placement of a drainage tube may be performed (cholecystostomy).

Clinical scenario

- A 58-year-old man presented with acute abdominal pain, pyrexia and RUQ tenderness. He had undergone laparoscopic cholecystectomy 4 years earlier. CT showed a round dense object in the subhepatic space surrounded by a rim or soft-tissue density (**Figure 6.4**).

- This is a dropped gallstone and is common during laparoscopic cholecystectomy. The incidence of gallbladder perforation is 15–30%, whereas the incidence of spillage of gallstone is approximately 10–12% during laparoscopic cholecystectomies. A dropped gallstone may serve as a nidus of infection and abscess formation. Patients may not present until several years after the original surgery.

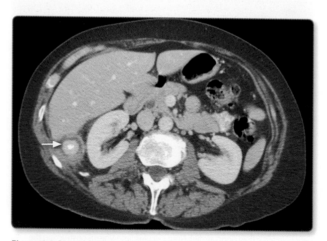

Figure 6.4 Dropped gallstone (arrow) with surrounding abscess in the subhepatic region at the level of the lower pole of the kidney.

6.2 Cholangiocarcinoma

Cholangiocarcinoma arises from the bile duct epithelium. These tumours can involve the intra- or extrahepatic bile ducts. Cholangiocarcinomas are the second most common primary liver tumours after hepatocellular carcinomas. Patients may present with painless jaundice, enlarged liver, anorexia or abdominal pain.

Key facts

- There is increased risk of developing cholangiocarcinoma in patients with ulcerative colitis (10 times) and those with primary sclerosing cholangitis, chronic biliary tract infections or inflammation (e.g. clonorchis, stones)
- Cholangiocarcinoma affecting the liver hilum at the junction of the left and right main hepatic ducts is termed 'Klatskin tumour'.

Radiological findings

Cholangiocarcinomas can be infiltrative, mass-forming or intraductal polypoid tumours, so radiological findings reflect these three types of tumour involvement.

US Biliary dilatation is the most common indirect sign of a cholangiocarcinoma, with the abrupt change in ductal diameter indicating the site of the tumour. Mass-forming cholangiocarcinomas may be hypoechoic, hyperechoic or of mixed echogenicity depending on their size and cellularity. Ductal or infiltrating cancers are difficult to detect on ultrasonography.

Percutaneous transhepatic cholangiogram (PTC). This typically shows strictures in the bile ducts (**Figure 6.5**). PTC involves injection of a contrast agent into a bile duct and then radiographs are taken.

CT On CT most cholangiocarcinomas remain hypodense during the arterial and portal venous phases and show enhancement during the delayed phase (5 min post-contrast) (**Figure 6.6**).

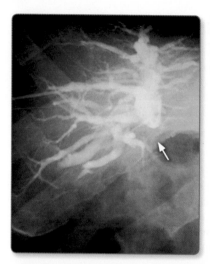

Figure 6.5 Percutaneous transhepatic cholangiography showing dilated bile ducts (arrow) with obstruction at the hilum.

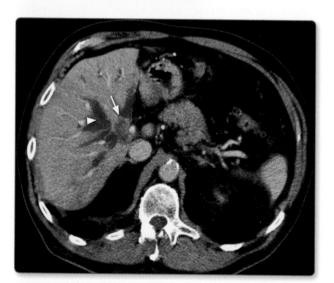

Figure 6.6 CT scan showing a round, enhancing lesion in the bile duct (arrow) causing bile duct obstruction and dilatation (arrowhead). Cholangiocarcinomas of the hilum are commonly termed 'Klatskin tumours'.

MRI MRI, along with MR cholangiopancreatography (MRCP – using MRI to visualise pancreatic and bile ducts non-invasively), is best for the assessment of intraductal lesions, because of its superior contrast resolution. On MRI relative to the liver parenchyma, intraductal lesions appear hypo- to isointense on T1-weighted and hypointense on T2-weighted images. MRCP can further complement contrast-enhanced MRI in depicting the site of ductal obstruction and associated upstream biliary dilatation.

Key imaging findings
A. Bile duct dilatation
B. Mass lesions on US or CT/MRI
C. Delayed contrast enhancement on CT
D. Strictures in the bile ducts on MRCP

Treatment
Surgical resection or liver transplantation. Radiological biliary stenting may be done to alleviate symptoms and obstruction.

6.3 Cirrhosis

Cirrhosis of the liver is a chronic, diffuse disease of the liver parenchyma causing fibrosis, hepatocytic necrosis and regenerative nodular changes. The cumulative 5-year risk of developing hepatocellular carcinoma is 10–15% in patients with cirrhosis. The most common causes are viral hepatitis and alcoholic abuse. Other causes include drug-induced cirrhosis, cardiac cirrhosis and liver steatosis.

Key facts
- Cirrhosis may be broadly classified morphologically as micronodular, macronodular or mixed type
- Although many aetiological factors cause cirrhosis, the end result is the destruction of liver parenchyma, fibrosis and formation of regenerative parenchymal nodules.

Radiological findings
The classic appearance is that of atrophy of the right lobe and

hypertrophy of the left lobe of the liver with a nodular contour (**Figure 6.7**). US, CT or MRI of the liver may show multiple nodules (**Figure 6.8**). Ascites is a common finding. In cases with concomitant portal hypertension, there is enlargement of the portal vein (>13 mm) with multiple enlarged collateral vessels. These collateral vessels are typically seen at the falciform ligament, around the gastro-oesophageal junction and the splenic hilum. MRI is best suited to detect nodules and hepatocellular carcinoma on a background of cirrhotic liver. Dysplastic nodules are hyperintense on T1-weighted and hypointense on T2-weighted scans compared with the liver parenchyma. Hepatocellular carcinoma nodules are hyperintense on T2-weighted scans and show increased contrast enhancement.

Key imaging findings
A. Atrophy of right lobe
B. Nodular contour of the liver
C. Multiple nodules within the liver
D. Distended portal vein with collaterals and ascites

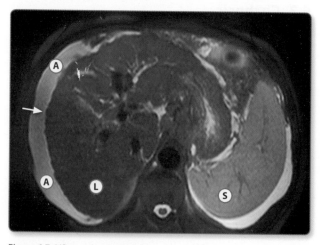

Figure 6.7 MR scan showing nodular outline of the liver (arrow) with surrounding ascites Ⓐ. Ⓛ liver, Ⓢ spleen.

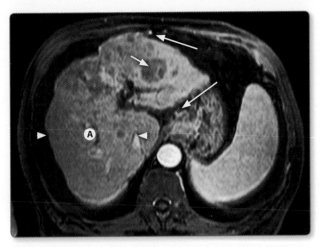

Figure 6.8 MR scan showing a cirrhotic liver with multiple enhancing nodules (short arrow). Note enlarged collateral vessels at the falciform ligament and around the gastro-oesophageal junction (long arrows). (A) Atrophy of the right lobe is seen (between arrowheads).

Treatment

In advanced cases liver transplantation may be required. Management is usually symptom based and medications such as steroids, a high-protein diet and alcohol abstinence are used.

6.4 Gallbladder cancer

Gallbladder cancer is an epithelial neoplasm, which arises from the gallbladder mucosa. It carries a poor prognosis. Patients usually present with abdominal pain, jaundice and weight loss. A non-tender mass may often be palpated in the right upper quadrant.

Key facts

- Gallbladder cancer is three times more frequent in women and average age of presentation is 70 years
- Most patients (>75%) also have associated gallstones

- Porcelain (completely calcified) gallbladder is particularly prone to malignant transformation and up to 25% of people with this condition have cancer
- Over 90% of these tumours are adenocarcinomas.

Radiological findings

US This is usually the first examination, with the most common finding (65%) being that of a hypoechoic mass filling or replacing the lumen of the gallbladder with invasion of the surrounding liver parenchyma (**Figure 6.9**). Other findings include focal thickening of the gallbladder wall (20%) or a polypoid mass in the lumen (25%). As gallbladder stones are often associated with cancer, echogenic shadowing produced by stones from within the mass ('contained stone' sign) is highly suggestive of cancer.

CT Usually hypodense on unenhanced CT, but hypervascular foci of enhancement (viable tumour tissue) are seen on contrast-enhanced scans. Most tumours demonstrate ill-defined

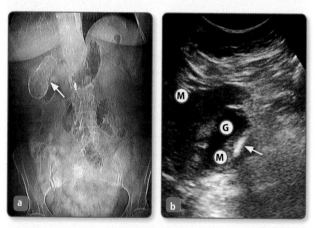

Figure 6.9 (a) Radiograph shows a porcelain gallbladder with calcification within the gallbladder wall (arrow). (b) US image showing gallbladder cancer as a soft tissue mass (M) with contained echogenic stone (arrow). (G) gallbladder.

areas of involvement of surrounding liver, with the clear fat planes between the gallbladder and liver being obliterated (**Figure 6.10**). Biliary obstruction at the level of the porta hepatis and lymph node metastasis are frequent associated findings.

Key imaging findings

A. Hypoechoic mass replacing gallbladder lumen on US
B. Contains stone sign
C. Infiltration of gallbladder bed and liver
D. Obstruction of bile ducts

Treatment

Gallbladder cancer has a poor prognosis, especially as early diagnosis is difficult. Early tumours may be resected surgically whereas advanced tumours are treated by chemo- and radiotherapy.

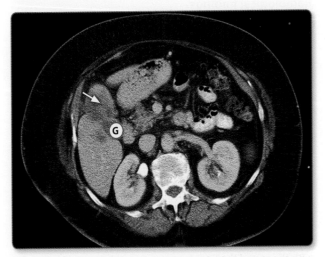

Figure 6.10 CT scan showing advanced gallbladder cancer with irregular infiltration of the liver (arrow). **G** gallbladder.

6.5 Haemangiomas

Haemangiomas are benign tumours of the liver comprising multiple, large vascular channels in a thin fibrous stroma. They are common and occur in 10% of the adult population.

Key facts

- Small haemangiomas are asymptomatic, whereas large lesions may cause abdominal pain and rarely may rupture or become secondarily infected
- More common in females
- Frequently located in the subcapsular region of the right lobe of the liver
- Haemangiomas are associated with several clinical syndromes, including Klippel–Trenaunay–Weber syndrome, Osler–Rendu–Weber disease and von Hippel–Lindau disease.

Radiological findings

Haemangiomas are usually detected incidentally on US or CT/MRI. The pathognomonic feature of haemangiomas is peripheral, nodular enhancement of CT and MRI with delayed contrast filling of the centre.

US Haemangiomas typically appear as rounded, hyperechoic (brighter than the normal liver) lesions. They are usually located in the subcapsular location. Posterior to the lesion, acoustic enhancement may be seen (**Figure 6.11**) as a bright band of echoes behind the lesion.

CT Haemangiomas are typically hypodense (compared with the liver), cyst-like lesions on non-contrast scans. On arterial phase imaging (30 s after contrast injection) haemangiomas show peripheral, nodular enhancement. On the portal phase (60 s) and delayed imaging (5 min) there is slow, filling in of contrast in the centre of the lesion until it is completely isodense with the rest of the liver.

MRI On T2-weighted scans, haemangiomas appear very bright (hyperintense) with the brightness increasing on heavier T2 weighting. This is termed the 'light bulb' sign. Contrast enhancement of the periphery with delayed filling in is again observed after contrast injection as on CT (**Figure 6.12**).

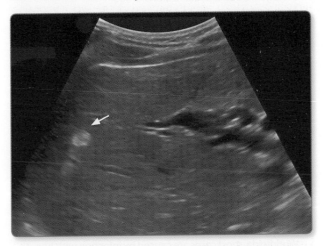

Figure 6.11 US scan showing a haemangioma seen as a rounded echogenic lesion (arrow) in the liver. Note the subtle posterior band of acoustic enhancement (brightness).

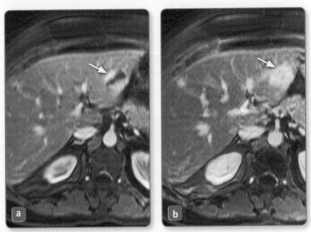

Figure 6.12 MR scan of haemangioma or arterial and portal phases showing peripheral, nodular enhancement with filling in on the portal phase (arrows).

Key imaging findings

A. Echogenic, subcapsular lesions on US
B. High signal intensity on MRI – 'light bulb sign'
C. Peripheral enhancement on arterial images
D. Delayed, central 'filling in' with contrast

Treatment

No treatment is required for small haemangiomas. Large haemangiomas causing symptoms may require excision.

6.6 Hepatitis

Hepatitis is an acute inflammation of the liver caused by viruses, drugs or excessive alcohol intake. The diagnosis of hepatitis is made by the combination of clinical history, serology, liver function tests and histology obtained by liver biopsy.

Key facts

- Worldwide, most cases are caused by infection with hepatitis viruses (A, B, C, D or E)
- Hepatocellular carcinomas occur in many patients with chronic viral infections.

Radiological findings

US there is hepatosplenomegaly with the liver showing decreased echogenicity. The portal triads appear more echogenic and, together with low echoes from the rest of the liver, this forms the 'starry sky' appearance (**Figure 6.13**). The gallbladder wall is thickened. Periportal hypoechoic tracks may be present due to hepatocytic oedema, which can manifest chronically as loss of definition of the portal triads.

MRI Periportal oedema is seen as a bright signal. MRI is very useful in chronic cases because it has high sensitivity in the detection of hepatocellular carcinoma. In alcoholic hepatitis there is marked loss of signal on out-of-phase MR scans due to fatty infiltration.

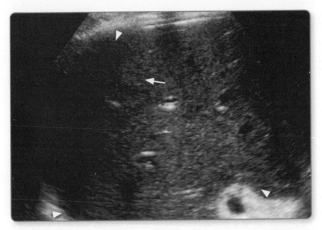

Figure 6.13 US scan showing an enlarged liver (arrowheads) with a diffuse speckled appearance in a patient with hepatitis. This is termed the 'starry sky appearance' (arrow).

Key imaging findings

A. Hepatosplenomegaly
B. Starry sky appearance
C. Periportal oedema
D. Loss of signal on out-of-phase MRI in alcoholic hepatitis

Treatment

No specific treatment is required for acute viral hepatitis. Cessation of alcohol should be encouraged for alcoholic hepatitis.

6.7 Hepatocellular carcinoma

Hepatocellular carcinoma (HCC) is the most common primary tumour of the liver. It is often a complication of cirrhosis and can be single or multifocal, with the overall incidence being 2.5% per year in patients with known cirrhosis. Patients may present with weight loss, pain, ascites, paraneoplastic syndrome or hepatomegaly.

Key facts

- There may be elevation of α-fetoprotein levels and altered liver function tests
- Most cases arise in cirrhotic livers due to chronic hepatitis B or C virus (HBV/HCV) infection or alcoholism
- HCCs are also associated with Wilson's disease, haemochromatosis and $α_1$-antitripsin deficiency.

Radiological findings

CT The pathognomonic finding is that of a large heterogeneous tumour with portal vein thrombosis. HCCs are predominantly hypodense masses on CT and may contain central areas of necrosis (hypodense, non-enhancing areas). As these tumours have a predominant arterial blood supply, they are best visualised on arterial phase imaging (**Figure 6.14**). Small tumours may be missed if only portal phase imaging is employed.

MRI This is the best method for detection of HCCs, particularly in cirrhotic livers. HCCs also show high signal on T1-weighted images, which is uncommon in other lesions (**Figure 6.15**). A thin tumour capsule is visible in most patients on MRI (**Figure 6.16**).

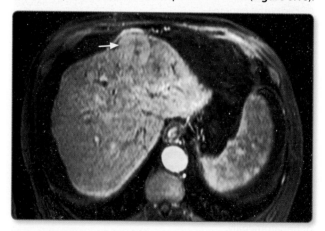

Figure 6.14 Enhancing lesion (arrow) on a background of cirrhotic liver suggestive of an hepatocellular carcinoma.

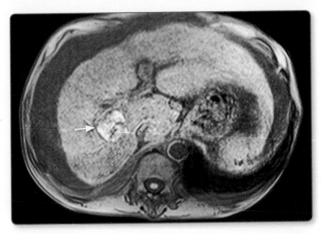

Figure 6.15 Axial T1-weighted MRI showing high signal (arrow) within a lesion in a cirrhotic liver.

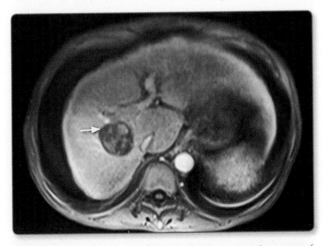

Figure 6.16 Axial postcontrast image showing heterogeneous enhancement of tumour within a thin capsule (arrow).

Key imaging findings

A. Heterogeneous density mass lesion on CT
B. Portal venous thrombosis
C. Thin capsule on MRI
D. High signal on T1-weighted MRI

Treatment

Surgical resection. Radiofrequency ablation (RFA) of tumours <3 cm under CT or US guidance.

6.8 Hepatic metastases

Metastases are the most common tumours of the liver. They may present with RUQ pain, mass or jaundice.

Key facts

Metastases may be hypervascular or hypovascular, which on contrast CT are seen as hyperdense or hypodense lesions.

Radiological findings

Liver metastases are typically seen as multiple, rounded lesions in the liver on US, CT or MRI. Hypervascular metastases arise from primary thyroid, renal, some breast and endocrine cancers. Melanoma metastases are also hypervascular. These metastases appear hyperdense on the arterial phase CT or MR scans (**Figure 6.17**).

Most, however, are hypovascular arising from lung, breast, gastrointestinal (GI) tract, pancreatic primaries or lymphoma and are hypodense on CT and hypointense on post-contrast MRI (**Figures 6.18** and **6.19**). Calcification may be seen in metastases from colloid colon cancers. Cystic (non-enhancing) metastases may be seen with breast primaries, whereas haemorrhagic (containing blood–fluid levels) lesions may be seen with melanoma metastases.

MRI Metastases are usually hypointense on T1-weighted and hyperintense on T2-weighted scans.

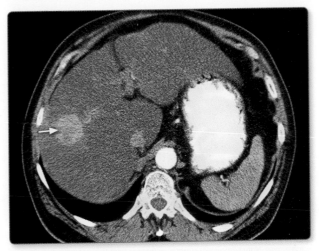

Figure 6.17 CT scan of liver metastasis from a hypervascular carcinoid tumour enhancing (arrow) in the arterial phase.

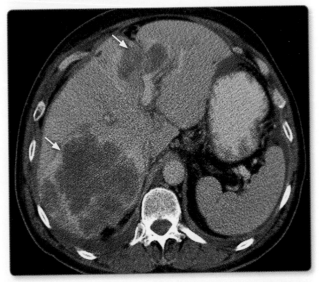

Figure 6.18 Colorectal metastasis appearing as hypodense lesions (arrows) on a CT scan.

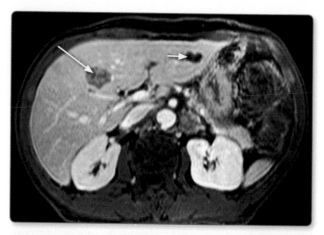

Figure 6.19 Colorectal disease metastasis seen as hypointense lesion on MRI (long arrow). Note completely cystic hypointense benign cyst (short arrow).

Key imaging findings

A. Hypodense or hyperdense, multiple, rounded lesions
B. High signal intensity on T2-weighted MRI
C. Calcification seen in some colon cancer metastases
D. Cystic metastases may be seen from breast primaries.

Treatment

Treatment depends on the primary cancer. Hepatic resection or radiofrequency ablation may be carried out for small lesions located within a single lobe.

6.9 Pancreatic cancer

Pancreatic cancers are mostly adenocarcinomas arising from the ductal epithelium. Smoking, diabetes and chronic pancreatitis are reported risk factors. Sixty per cent are cancers of the pancreatic head and can present with painless jaundice, weight loss and epigastric mass. Cancers of the body may spread in the retroperitoneum, causing pain due to involvement of the splanchnic nerves.

Key facts

- Gene mutations associated with pancreatic cancer have been well established, and include *KRAS2* (80–95%), *CDKN2* (85–98%), *p53* (50%) and *Smad4* (55%)
- Most patients present with advanced, non-resectable disease
- Migratory thrombophlebitis is characteristic of pancreatic cancer and is termed 'Trousseau's sign'

Radiological findings

Barium examination A 'reversed 3' configuration of the duodenum is observed, termed the 'reverse 3' or 'Frostberg sign'. This is due to the mass effect created by pancreatic head enlargement, and can also result from chronic pancreatitis.

US Pancreatic cancers appear as hypoechoic, irregular masses seen with associated dilatation of the pancreatic and biliary ducts – 'double-duct sign'; there is simultaneous dilatation of both pancreatic and common bile ducts.

CT Best suited for the diagnosis and staging of pancreatic cancers. Most adenocarcinomas are hypovascular, therefore appearing as hypodense lesions on CT (**Figure 6.20**). Infiltration

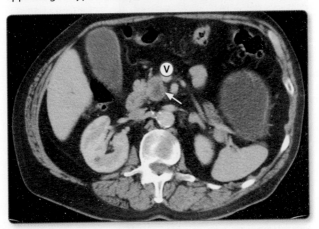

Figure 6.20 CT scan showing pancreatic tumour as a hypodense lesion (arrow) within the pancreatic head. Ⓥ superior mesenteric vein.

of adjacent structures, lymphadenopathy and the presence of distant metastasis can also be evaluated for suitability of resection. The 'double-duct sign' seen on imaging is pathognomonic of pancreatic cancers (**Figure 6.21**). Vascular invasion is seen as a cuff of soft tissue surrounding or narrowing the superior mesenteric blood vessels (**Figure 6.22**).

ERCP and MRCP On endoscopic cholangiopacreatography (ERCP) or MRCP an irregular appearing stricture (as opposed to a smooth narrowing) may be seen. ERCP uses endoscopy and fluoroscopy to diagnose biliary and pancreatic duct problems.

Key imaging findings
A. Irregular hypodense or hypoechoic mass lesion
B. 'Reverse 3' sign
C. Double-duct sign
D. Stricture on MRCP or ERCP

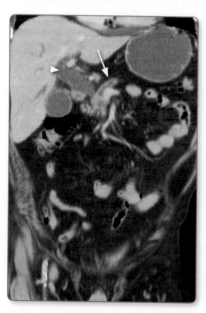

Figure 6.21 Pancreatic tumour causing dilation of the common bile duct (arrowhead) and pancreatic duct (arrow) – forming the 'double duct sign'.

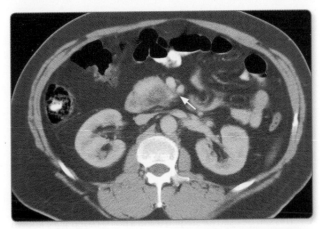

Figure 6.22 CT scan of pancreatic tumour with vascular involvement seen as soft-tissue cuffing and tethering of the superior mesenteric vein and artery (arrow).

Treatment

Small tumours can be excised or a pancreaticoduodenectomy (Whipple's operation) performed. Advanced tumours require chemotherapy. Biliary stents may be placed radiologically for palliation of obstruction.

6.10 Pancreatitis

Inflammation of the pancreatic gland usually occurs due to blockage of the pancreatic duct, causing release of pancreatic enzymes into the bloodstream. Patients may present with acute onset of abdominal pain, nausea, vomiting, abdominal distension, hypotension or shock. Flank ecchymosis (large bruising; Grey Turner's sign), or periumbilical bruising and oedema (Cullen's sign) may also be seen.

Key facts

The common causes of pancreatitis are blockage of the duct by stones, tumours or inflammation related to alcohol abuse.

Radiological findings

Radiograph This may show ileus with loss of the psoas margins. In acute-on-chronic pancreatitis, calcification may be seen. Inflammation can also involve the splenic flexure of the colon as it travels along the pancreatic tail and up the left phrenicocolic ligament, appearing as a cut-off of the colonic gas shadow in the left upper quadrant (the 'colon cut-off' sign) (**Figure 6.23**).

US Gallstones are a common cause best seen on US. Stones in the common bile duct (CBD) may be missed due to overlying gas and inflammation of the pancreas. In such cases MRCP can allow accurate assessment. The pancreas is enlarged and there is surrounding inflammation.

CT This can be used for staging using a point-based scale known as Balthazar staging, which takes into account pancreatic necrosis, cysts, abscesses and collections. Postpancreatitic complications include formation of pancreatic pseudocysts (enzymes, blood and necrotic tissues), portal venous thrombosis, haemorrhage and abscess formation (**Figures 6.24** and **6.25**). There is extensive calcification of the pancreas in chronic pancreatitis (**Figure 6.26** and see **Figure 3.7**), with distortion and cystic dilatation of the pancreatic duct (**Figure 6.27**). This is due to the deposition of

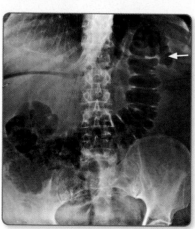

Figure 6.23 Radiograph showing abrupt cut-off of the colonic gas shadow at the splenic flexure (arrow) – the 'colon cut-off' sign.

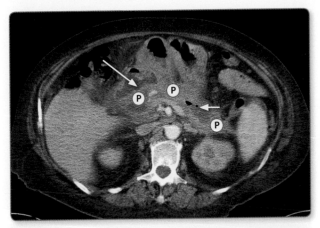

Figure 6.24 CT scan showing extensive inflammation (long arrow) with streaking and loss of the fat planes around the pancreas (P). A small abscess containing gas is also present within the pancreatic tail (short arrow).

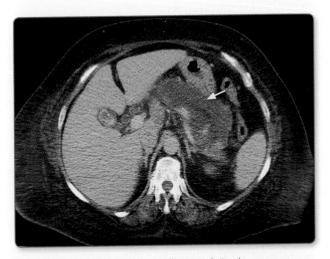

Figure 6.25 CT scan showing a cystic collection replacing the pancreas consistent with a pseudocyst (arrow). Note hyperdense elements within the cyst, which are due to haemorrhage.

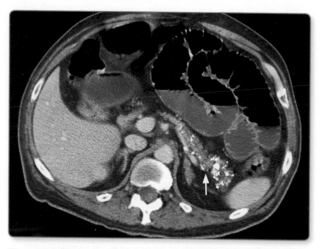

Figure 6.26 CT scan showing speckled calcification in the pancreas (arrow) secondary to chronic pancreatitis.

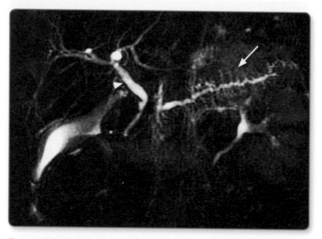

Figure 6.27 MR cholangiopancreatography showing dilated and ectatic pancreatic duct (arrow) with dilatation of the side branches. These findings are indicative of chronic pancreatitis. Common bile duct (arrowhead).

proteinaceous and inflammatory material in the pancreatic ducts which forms protein plugs that subsequently calcify.

Key imaging findings

A. Colon cut-off sign
B. Pancreatic enlargement and inflammation
C. Cystic collections
D. Ascites and left-sided pleural effusions

Treatment

Symptomatic and supportive treatment.

6.11 Portal hypertension

Portal hypertension (PH) signifies an increased pressure gradient (>8 mmHg) between the portal and hepatic (systemic) venous systems. The most common cause of PH is liver cirrhosis. PH can cause ascites, splenomegaly and distended veins in the portacaval anastomoses/collaterals (oesophageal/gastric, anorectal and umbilical varices). Oesophageal varices are particularly at risk of bleeding, potentially causing life-threatening haematemesis.

Key facts

- PH occurs when flow to the portal vein is impeded and blood has to travel through collaterals to reach the systemic circulation
- PH may be extrahepatic (i.e. splenic vein obstruction), hepatic (at sinusoidal level such as caused by cirrhosis) or posthepatic (i.e. obstruction of blood flow between the hepatic veins and inferior vena cava such as in Budd–Chiari syndrome)

Radiological findings

US US and Doppler are essential to diagnose PH. In established PH the diameter of the portal vein is >13 mm (**Figure 6.28**), and reversed flow is detectable (pathognomonic). Other findings include the presence of collateral vessels such as the coronary veins (>5 mm) and the umbilical vein in the ligamentum teres.

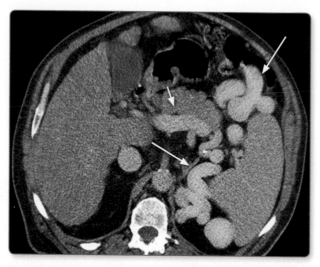

Figure 6.28 CT scan showing multiple large collateral vessels around the spleen and splenorenal region (long arrows) in a patient with portal hypertension. Note enlarged portal vein (short arrow) posterior to the pancreas.

Other secondary signs seen on US include splenomegaly, ascites, and splenorenal and umbilical collaterals.

Key imaging findings

A. Dilated portal vein >13 mm in diameter
B. Hepatofugal blood flow
C. Presence of collateral veins
D. Ascites

Treatment

Treatment is by creating shunts between the portal and systemic veins (such as hepatic veins) to divert blood flow. Shunts can be fashioned surgically or intrahepatic shunts can be created using a radiological procedures (transjugular intrahepatic portal shunts or TIPS).

6.12 Trauma – hepatosplenic injury

The liver or spleen is commonly injured by blunt abdominal trauma, and there is often associated injury to the ribs and kidneys. Patients present with a history of trauma, flank pain and hypotension from blood loss.

Key facts

Rupture of the spleen may occur after relatively minor trauma in patients with massive splenomegaly secondary to infections (e.g. due to malaria), haematological causes or tumours.

Radiological findings

Clinical insight

Haemoperitoneum is best seen in the hepatorenal pouch where small amounts of fluid (<5 ml) can be detected

US This shows lacerations as linear hypoechoic areas within the spleen or liver. Fresh haemorrhage imparts an echogenic or heterogeneous appearance (**Figure 6.29**). Pericapsular fluid collections may be seen (**Figure 6.29**). In up

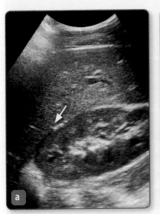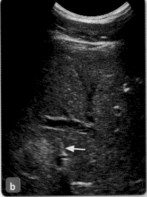

Figure 6.29 Hepatosplenic trauma: haemoperitoneum manifesting as small crescent of hypoechoic fluid in the hepatorenal pouch (arrow); haemorrhagic contusion in the liver seen as an irregular hyperechoic area (arrow).

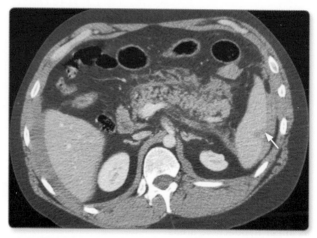

Figure 6.30 Splenic contusion seen as a focal area of non-enhancement (arrow). Note that fluid around the spleen is dense compared with fluid around the liver. This density suggests the presence of blood (haemoperitoneum).

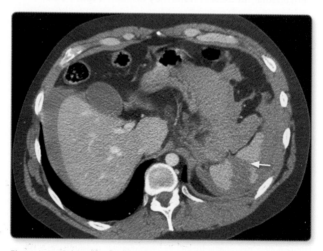

Figure 6.31 Splenic fracture is seen as complete disruption (arrow) of the spleen with non-enhancement and surrounding fluid.

to 20% of cases adequate examination may not be possible due to rib fractures and tenderness.

CT This shows irregular hypodense areas corresponding to lacerations (**Figure 6.30**). Subcapsular haematomas are demonstrated as crescentic collections around the spleen. Splenic fractures are seen as linear non-enhancing areas traversing the width of the spleen (**Figure 6.31**).

Key imaging findings
A. Linear, irregular hypoechoic areas in the spleen
B. Pericapsular fluid collections
C. Crescentic collections around the spleen
D. Irregular non-enhancing areas traversing the spleen

Treatment
Most splenic injuries are treated conservatively.

Paediatrics

Paediatric abdominal disorders may have an acute presentation early in life. Usually such disorders are due to congenital disorders and include diseases such as hypertrophic pyloric stenosis. Congenital disorders may be detected on antenatal US. Tumours such as neuroblastomas and nephroblastomas are also common in young patients. It is important to recognise abnormal signs on abdominal imaging to detect pathologies because young patients quite often are not able to provide adequate clinical history.

7.1 Cryptorchidism

Cryptorchidism is the failure of testicular descent into the scrotal sac. The undescended testes may lie anywhere along the line of the ureter and spermatic cord, although the most common location is at or below the inguinal canal.

Key facts

- Undescended testes are common in preterm infants
- There is a high risk of malignant change in undescended testes (4–40 times that in the general population)
- The cause is unknown but may be related to higher body temperature within the abdominal cavity rather than the scrotal sac leading to malignant change.

Radiological findings

US This is the procedure of choice in the diagnosis of cryptorchidism. The scrotal sac is empty (**Figure 7.1**) and the undescended testicle is seen as an ovoid structure at or below the inguinal canal. Usually the ectopic testicle is smaller and more hypoechoic than the normal testicle.

CT/MRI If the undescended testis is not located in the inguinal region, CT or MRI is useful in locating the abdominal testis.

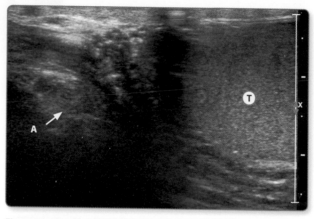

Figure 7.1 US scan of the scrotum showing an empty scrotal sac in a patient with undescended testes (arrow A). (T) Normal left-sided testicle is present.

Key imaging findings

A. Empty scrotal sac
B. Testicle in the region of the inguinal canal
C. Smaller and more hypoechoic than normal testes
D. CT used for locating abdominal testis.

Treatment

Orchidopexy.

7.2 Hypertrophic pyloric stenosis

Hypertrophic pyloric stenosis is the most common cause of neonatal upper gastrointestinal (GI) tract obstruction. Presentation is most commonly between 4 and 6 weeks of age with projectile vomiting and epigastric mass.

Key facts

The obstruction is caused by hypertrophy of the pyloric muscle and is much more common in boys (four times more common in first-born boys).

Radiological findings

US This has a key role in diagnosis. The pylorus appears thickened (>4 mm is considered diagnostic) as a concentric hypoechoic ring with few echoes centrally (**Figure 7.2**). Distended stomach with hyperperistalsis may also be present. Some studies have shown that the length of the pyloric canal >17 mm is a more accurate predictor of this disease than just muscle thickness.

Barium examination A thin, single or double track of contrast is seen outlining the pyloric canal.

Key imaging findings
A. Muscle thickness >4 mm
B. Pyloric canal length >17 mm
C. Double-track sign on barium examination
D. Distended stomach

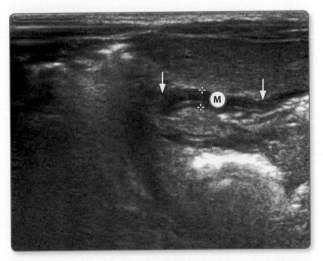

Figure 7.2 US scan showing hypertrophic pyloric muscle, seen as a thickened elongated muscular structure (between arrows). ⓜ Pyloric muscle mass is thickened (between callipers).

Treatment

Treatment is by surgical division of the pyloric muscle known as Ramstedt's procedure.

7.3 Intussusception

Intussusception is caused by a segment of bowel (intussusceptum) invaginating or telescoping into its adjacent segment (intussuscipiens). The most common location is the ileocaecal region. Patients commonly present with abdominal pain and vomiting. The classic triad of acute abdominal pain, currant-jelly stools or haematochezia, and an abdominal mass is present in less than 50% of children.

Key facts

- Intussusception is the second most common cause of acute abdomen in infants and children after appendicitis
- This condition usually occurs in children aged between 6 months and 2 years
- It is most often idiopathic and caused by lymphoid hyperplasia
- Intussusception is rare is adults and, when present, is often associated with an underlying lesion (neoplasm).

Radiological findings

Radiograph Findings of bowel obstruction such as bowel dilatation and multiple fluid levels may be seen on radiographs. A crescent of air may be present around the intussusceptum, creating the 'claw sign' often seen in the right hypochondrium (**Figure 7.3**).

Barium examination A pathognomonic 'coiled spring' appearance is caused by barium trapped between two segments of bowel telescoped within each other.

US This is the first-line investigation in children and infants. Typically a 'target' (transverse scans) or 'trilaminar' or 'pitchfork'

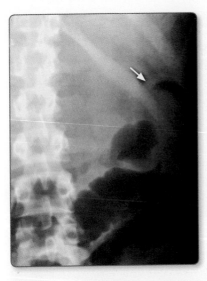

Figure 7.3 Radiograph showing a crescent of air in the left upper quadrant forming the 'claw sign' (arrow).

(longitudinal scans) appearance is seen, caused by the presence of bowel within bowel in the intussusception (**Figure 7.4**).

CT The target appearance is again seen, consisting of circular hypodense areas (mesenteric fat) alternating with hyperdense areas (bowel wall).

Key imaging findings
A. Claw sign on radiographs
B. 'Coiled spring' appearance
C. Trilaminar or pitchfork appearance on US
D. Target sign on US and CT

Treatment
In adults, surgery may be necessary. In children pneumatic or hydrostatic reduction of the intussusception is often employed by instilling air/fluid through the rectum.

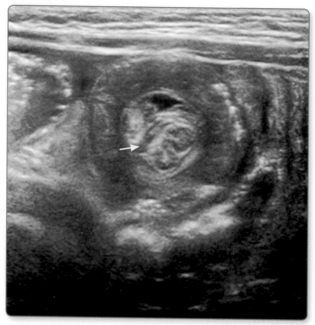

Figure 7.4 US scan showing intussusception as concentric layers of bowel within bowel or target pattern (arrow).

7.4 Necrotising enterocolitis

Necrotising enterocolitis (NEC) is a significant cause of morbidity and mortality, particularly in preterm babies and may occur in 1–8% of all neonatal admissions. Clinically babies develop bloody diarrhoea, abdominal distension and positive blood cultures.

Key facts

The causative factor of NEC appears to be intestinal mucosal injury (the exact aetiology in unknown, but is most probably due to ischaemic insult in preterm babies), followed by invasion and spread of bacteria through the breach.

Radiological findings

Radiograph This shows dilated bowel loops. The pathognomonic hallmark of NEC is the presence of pneumatosis intestinalis (gas in the bowel wall), seen as linear tracks of air in the wall of the intestine (**Figure 7.5**). Gas may also be present in the branches of the mesenteric vessels and the portal vein (**Figure 7.6**). Gas in the portal vein is seen as branching areas of lucency in the periphery of the liver. Pneumatosis and portal venous gas may be best demonstrated on radiographs taken in the left-side-down decubitus position. Strictures may form, particularly in the colon after medical or surgical treatment.

Key imaging findings

A. Distended bowel loops
B. Pneumatosis intestinalis
C. Strictures
D. Portal venous gas

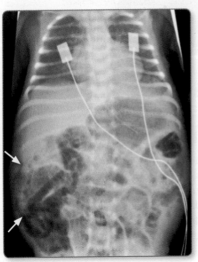

Figure 7.5 Distended bowel loops with pneumatosis (gas within bowel wall) (arrows) seen in a child with necrotising enterocolitis.

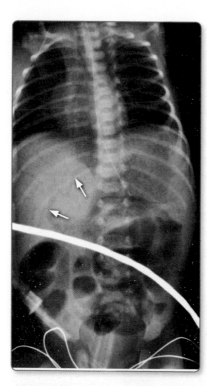

Figure 7.6 Distended bowel loops with portal venous gas seen as linear branching structures in the liver (arrows).

Treatment
Medical treatment and parenteral nutrition. Surgical treatment may be required in cases with perforation of the bowel.

7.5 Congenital renal anomalies

Congenital renal anomalies may be due to abnormality in location, number, fusion and form of the renal tract. These anomalies constitute up to 20–30% of all anomalies identified in the prenatal period. Common anomalies include fusion of kidneys (horseshoe kidney), unilateral renal agenesis, polycystic kidneys, renal or ureteric duplication, pelviureteric junction

(PUJ) obstruction and ureterocoeles. Presentation may be in antenatal or childhood period, whereas less serious malformations such as horseshoe kidney may remain asymptomatic.

Key facts

- Horseshoe kidneys are more prone to PUJ obstruction and renal calculi formation because the malformation leads to mechanical difficulty in urine flow
- Ureterocoeles are dilatations of the intramural portion of the ureter as it passes through the bladder wall; commonly associated with duplex kidneys.

Radiological findings

US/CT These show horseshoe kidneys having attachment or fusion along their lower poles (**Figure 7.7**). Crossed fused ectopia is when the kidneys are fused, with one in its normal position and the other across the midline. Polycystic kidneys (PKs) show

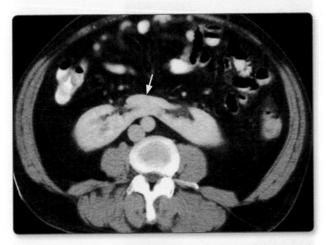

Figure 7.7 CT scan of a horseshoe kidney with fusion of the lower poles (arrow) across the midline. Note anteriorly oriented calyceal system, which is prone to stasis and stone formation.

multiple cysts of varying sizes in both kidneys. There are two types of PK: autosomal dominant polycystic kidney disease (ADPKD) and the less common autosomal recessive polycystic kidney disease (ARPKD). The cysts are numerous and result in massive enlargement of the kidneys. The disease can also affect the liver and pancreas. Renal and ureteric duplication are best seen on intravenous urography (IVU). Usually the duplex system is larger than the normal kidney. In cases with duplication of ureters, the ureter draining the upper pole of the kidney invariably has a lower insertion into the urinary bladder than that draining the lower pole (this inverse relationship is called the Weigert–Meyer law). Ectopic insertion of a ureter causes stenosis and saccular dilatation of the distal ureter (ureterocoele), resulting in a 'cobra-head' appearance on IVU (**Figure 7.8**).

Key imaging findings

A. Fusion of kidneys

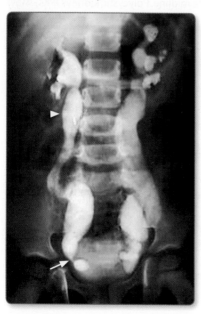

Figure 7.8 IVU showing bilateral ureterocoeles with proximal dilatation of ureters (arrowhead). The lower ends of the ureters have a bulbous, cobra head appearance (arrow).

B. Duplication of ureters
C. Cobra-head appearance
D. Multiple cysts in the kidneys

Treatment

Treatment depends on the underlying condition.

7.6 Common paediatric tumours – neuroblastomas

This is the most common extracranial solid tumour of childhood and in most cases arises from the adrenal glands. The annual incidence is about 600–650 new cases per year in the UK. Up to 50% of neuroblastoma cases occur in children aged <2 years. As the symptoms of the disease tend to be varied and vague, some two thirds of children are not diagnosed until the disease is widespread. Metastases are often the presenting feature, but other clinical signs include failure to thrive, weight loss, pyrexia and irritability.

Key facts

- It is a neuroendocrine tumour arising from the sympathetic nervous system
- Two thirds of neuroblastomas occur in the adrenal glands, whereas other locations include along the spine in the thorax or the abdomen

Radiological findings

Radiograph Fine stippled calcification may be seen on a radiograph with mass effect and displacement of bowel loops (**Figure 7.9**).

US On US the tumour is of mixed echogenicity and surrounds the aorta or inferior vena cava (IVC).

CT CT is needed for staging of these tumours and better demonstrates the full extent of the mass. It shows a mass surrounding the aorta and IVC with fine calcification (**Figure 7.10**).

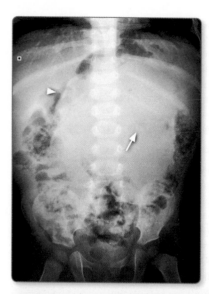

Figure 7.9 Radiograph showing a large soft-tissue mass (arrow) displacing bowel loops (arrowhead).

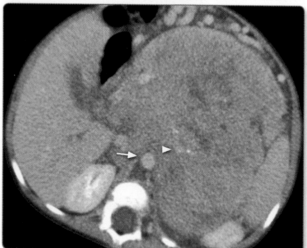

Figure 7.10 CT scan showing a large mass encasing the aorta (arrow) and stippled calcification (arrowhead). (Image courtesy of Dr G. Mann).

Extension into the neural foramina of the vertebral bodies may be present.

Key imaging findings

A. Mass with stippled calcification
B. Widening of paravertebral space
C. Mixed echo tumour surrounding the aorta and IVC
D. Extension into neural foramina

Treatment

Surgery with or without chemo- or radiotherapy.

7.7 Common paediatric tumours – Wilms' tumour

Wilms' tumour, also known as nephroblastoma, is the most common primary renal tumour in children and the peak incidence is in the group aged 3–4 years (0.8 cases per 100,000 children). The most common presentation is with an abdominal mass or distension (40%).

Key facts

- It is thought to arise from specialised cells in the embryo known as metanephric blastemas
- These cells are involved in the development of the kidneys and usually disappear at birth but, in many children with Wilms' tumour, they can still be found
- Wilms' tumours can be bilateral in 5% of cases and evaluation of both kidneys should be done as a rule
- It is associated with conditions such as aniridia, horseshoe kidneys and hemihypertrophy.

Radiological findings

Radiograph Radiographs may reveal a soft-tissue mass displacing bowel loops.

US This is usually the first investigation. Wilms' tumours appear as mass lesions arising from the kidney and typically have

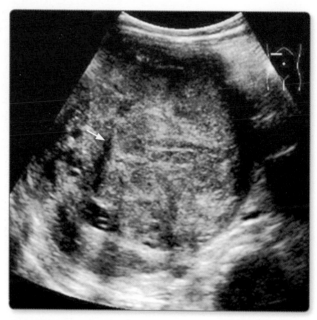

Figure 7.11 US scan showing a large heteroechoic lesion with low echo areas (arrow) in a child with an abdominal mass.

echogenic areas interspersed with low echo areas (**Figure 7.11**). Calcification is seen in up to 20% of cases and is arc or ring like in configuration (**Figure 7.12**). The lungs are the most common sites of metastases due to haematogenous spread.

Key imaging findings
A. Mass lesion with echogenic and low echo areas on US
B. Arc or ring-like calcification
C. Bilateral tumours on CT
D. Lung metastases

Treatment
Surgical excision.

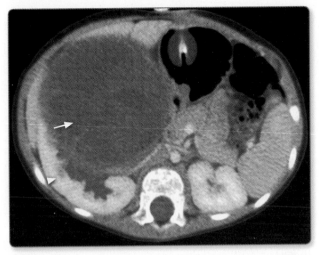

Figure 7.12 CT scan showing a large, predominantly hypodense mass (arrow) arising from the right kidney (arrowhead). (Image courtesy of Dr G. Mann).

7.8 VACTERL syndrome

The acronym VACTERL describes a constellation of congenital abnormalities that include vertebral anomalies, anorectal malformations, cardiac abnormalities, tracheo-oesophageal fistula or atresia, renal abnormalities and limb defects. The true frequency is difficult to estimate but has been suggested as 1.6 cases per 10,000 live births.

Key facts
- Of the above-mentioned anomalies, three of the seven should be present for a patient to be classified as having VACTERL syndrome
- Other abnormalities such as genital anomalies, thumb defects and cleft palate may also be present

Radiological findings

Anomalies may be detected by US on antenatal scanning. The most common cardiac abnormality is a ventricular septal defect (VSD). Anorectal atresia may be low or high (treatment depends on type of abnormality): in the low type, the bowel is normal up to the anal canal with a persistent anal membrane; whereas in the high type, distal bowel may be abnormal with fistulation into the genitourinary tract or abdominal wall (**Figure 7.13**). Due to bowel obstruction polyhydramnios (excessive amniotic fluid) or dilated bowel loops may be present on the antenatal scans. Patients with this syndrome usually have a single umbilical artery as well as abnormalities affecting the radius in the forearm (**Figure 7.14**).

Key imaging findings

A. Single umbilical artery
B. VSD
C. Anorectal atresia
D. Abnormalities of the radius

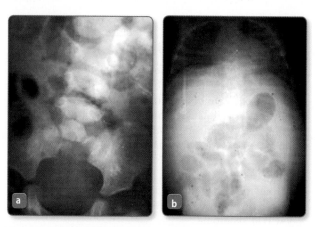

Figures 7.13 Radiographs showing (a) vertebral anomalies with absence of sacrum and (b) distended bowel with absent colon.

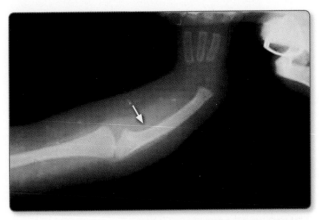

Figure 7.14 Radiograph showing the absence of the radius (arrow) in a child with VACTERL syndrome.

Treatment

Treatment depends on the type and severity of the abnormality present.

7.9 Vesicoureteric reflux

Vesicoureteric reflux (VUR) is retrograde flow of urine from the bladder into the ureters and kidneys and is associated with urinary tract infections (UTIs) and abnormal renal development such as renal atrophy. VUR is caused by abnormal bladder function (excessive muscular contractions) or orientation of the vesicoureteric opening that allows reflux. Patients often present with recurring UTIs and hydronephrosis.

Key facts

- VUR has a genetic element (up to 34% of children with it have an affected sibling) and usually presents in childhood, but occasionally may be seen in the antenatal US as hydronephrosis

- Reflux may cause renal scarring (associated with developing hypertension) and up to 30% of children with VUR may have renal cortical damage due to infections

Radiological findings

The classic appearance of VUR is based on IVU and micturating cystourethrography (MCU – filling bladder with contrast medium and taking radiographs). US may show hydronephrosis or scarring of kidneys. On MCU reflux may be seen into the ureters or kidneys (**Figure 7.15**). VUR is graded by radiology into five categories: grades 3–5 reflect reflux extending up to the kidney with resulting hydronephrosis (**Figure 7.16**). Radionuclide scans (99mTc–DMSA) are also used to check kidney function and look for scarring.

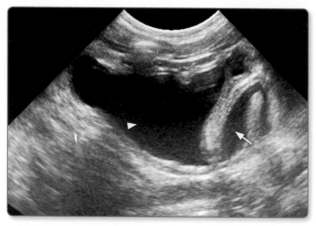

Figure 7.15 US scan showing hydronephrosis (arrowhead) with dilatation of the ureter (arrow) in a child with reflux.

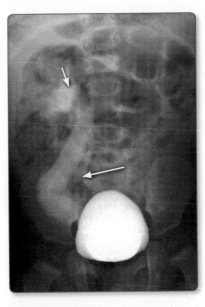

Figure 7.16 Micturating cystourethrogram shows Grade 5 reflux up to the kidneys (short arrow). Note the significant hydronephrosis and dilatation of the ureter (long arrow).

Key imaging findings
A. Hydronephrosis
B. Renal scarring
C. Ureteric dilatation
D. Reflux on MCU

Treatment
Treatment may be medical or surgical. Grades 1–3 often resolve with medical management by the age of 5. Prophylactic antibiotic therapy is carried out to prevent infections and renal damage. Surgical intervention with ureteric reimplantation may be carried out in persistent reflux and recurrent infections.

Key Insights & Notes

A. Fluid movement
B. Fluid handling
C. ...
D. Relevant skill set...

Treatment as...

Treatment may be medical or surgical. Grades 1-3 often require surgical management by the age of 5. Equally as important, the way learned out to prevent infection under the damage. Surgical intervention well outside family situation may be carried out if persistent reflux and recurrent infections...

Gynaecological disorders

Gynaecological disorders affect the female reproductive system which includes the uterus, ovaries and vagina. Common diseases include ovarian cysts, fibroids and inflammation of the fallopian tube. Some diseases such as ovarian cysts do not cause significant morbidity, whereas others such as ectopic pregnancy are known acute emergencies and can lead to massive blood loss and even death if not treated appropriately. US (transabdominal or transvaginal) is the primary modality used in evaluation of gynaecological disorders. In recent years, MRI has emerged as another important tool by virtue of its higher contrast resolution and ability to differentiate the solid, cystic and haemorrhagic tissues that characterise many gynaecological disorders.

8.1 Ectopic pregnancy

It is important to detect ectopic pregnancy early because it is a major cause of maternal mortality in the first trimester. Patients usually present with pain, inflammation and vaginal bleeding. Internal bleeding may cause pelvic and lower back pain and hypotension.

Key facts

Most ectopic pregnancies occur in the fallopian tubes but implantation can also occur in other sites such as the cervix, abdomen or ovaries.

Radiological findings

US Transvaginal US (TVUS) plays a major role in the detection or exclusion of ectopic pregnancy. The presence of a normal gestational sac within the uterus virtually excludes the diagnosis of ectopic pregnancy. TVUS can detect a normal sac earlier than abdominal US scans, when human β-chorionic gonadotrophin (β-hCG – serum marker produced by implanted egg) is between 500 and 1500 mIU/ml, versus >1500 mIU/ml for abdominal US. Doppler scans reveal high-velocity blood flow in the gestational sac of an ectopic pregnancy. Raised β-hCG in the absence of a gestational sac in the uterus is also compatible with diagnosis of an ectopic pregnancy.

US features of an ectopic pregnancy are the demonstration of a gestational sac outside the uterus (**Figures 8.1** and **8.2**). This usually appears as a rounded 10–30 mm cystic lesion (distended fallopian tube) in the adnexa, containing an echogenic, dense structure representing the gestational sac. The uterus may be moderately enlarged with a prominent endometrium echo. In a minority of patients the fetal heart may be seen within the gestational sac (after 5–6 weeks of gestational age). A ruptured ectopic pregnancy presents as a complex mass in the adnexa, consisting of echogenic blood products and fluid.

Key imaging findings

A. Empty uterus
B. Echogenic structure in a cystic lesion in the adnexa

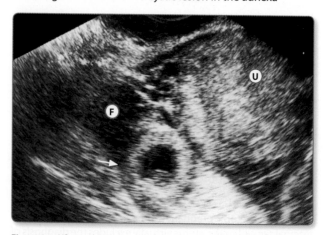

Figure 8.1 US scan showing ectopic pregnancy as cystic echogenic mass (arrow) in the adnexal region. Ⓕ free fluid, Ⓤ uterus.

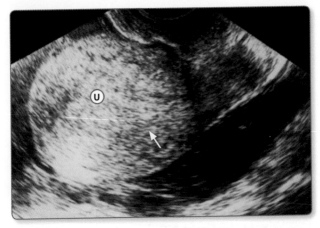

Figure 8.2 The uterus Ⓤ appears empty (arrow) in the same patient.

C. Fetal heartbeat
D. High-velocity Doppler flow

Treatment
Treatment is with surgical excision.

8.2 Endometriosis

Endometriosis is the occurrence of endometrial tissue in sites other than the uterine endometrial lining, commonly the rectouterine pouch (of Douglas), ovaries, rectovaginal septum and pelvic peritoneum. Endometriosis implants can also be seen at distant sites including the gastrointestinal (GI) tract, urinary system, hepatobiliary system, lungs and the skin. It can be associated with infertility, dysmenorrhoea, dyspareunia and abnormal menstrual bleeding.

Key facts
Endometriosis is now considered the most common cause of sterility in women aged >25 years.

Radiological findings
US TVUS is used for the initial evaluation. US is helpful in the

assessment of endometriotic cysts or larger implants. The typical appearance of ovarian endometriomas is of cystic masses with diffuse low-level homogeneous echoes (**Figure 8.3**). As endometriomas contain blood products from recurrent haemorrhage, these can produce a layered pattern or fluid–fluid/fluid–clot levels (**Figure 8.4**). Ovarian endometriomas are bilateral in a significant proportion of patients.

MRI Valuable in the diagnosis of superficial peritoneal implants and extraperitoneal lesions. Endometriomas are seen as cystic masses with high signal intensity on T1-weighted images and loss of signal intensity on T2-weighted images due to contained blood products. This 'shading sign' may occur in a graded form with higher to lower signal-intensity patterns, as a result of iron concentration from recurrent haemorrhage (see **Figure 8.4**).

Key imaging findings
A. Multiple or bilateral ovarian cysts
B. Fluid–fluid levels

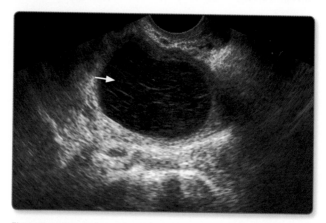

Figure 8.3 US scan of an endometrial cyst with low-level echoes (arrow) due to blood products.

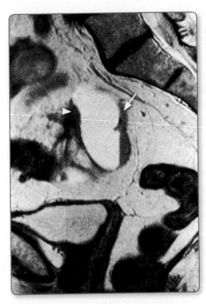

Figure 8.4 MR scan of an endometrial cyst showing a fluid level (arrow). Note dark, hypointense margins due to haemosiderin (arrowhead), known as the shading sign.

C. Shading sign on MRI
D. High signal on T1-weighed images due to haemorrhage.

Treatment

Treatment may be symptomatic to reduce pain. Hormonal treatment (e.g. progesterone) is used to shrink the size of endometriomas. Surgical treatment may be required for severe symptoms, infertility or involvement of other organs.

8.3 Fibroids

Also known as leiomyomas, these are benign tumours of the muscular layer of the uterus. Fibroids usually develop during a woman's reproductive years, because they are linked to oestrogen production. Most are asymptomatic; however, they can grow to cause heavy and painful menstruation, painful sexual intercourse or urinary symptoms.

Key facts

- Fibroids are the most common benign tumours in women and typically found during the middle/late reproductive years
- Fibroids can be located in the muscle wall (intramural), subserosal, submucosal, cervical or pedunculated.

Radiological findings

Radiograph Large fibroids may cause a soft-tissue shadow on radiographs. Up to 10% of fibroids may show dystrophic calcification, which is typically coarse and curvilinear in appearance (**Figure 8.5**). Occasionally a peripheral rim of calcification is present.

US US has high accuracy in fibroid detection. The typical appearance is of a lobular, well-defined mass with low-level echoes within the uterine body. Increased echogenicity may be seen in areas of degeneration or necrosis. Calcification within the fibroid causes dense shadowing on US.

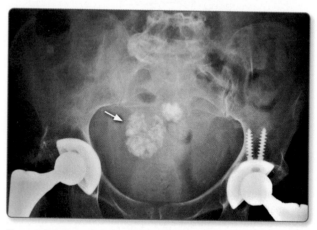

Figure 8.5 Radiograph showing a calcified fibroid (arrow) in the pelvis.

MRI MRI has greater accuracy than US in evaluating location, number and size of fibroids. The diagnostic finding is a sharply marginated mass which typically has lower signal intensity than the myometrium on T2-weighted images (**Figure 8.6**).

Key imaging findings

A. Location within the uterus
B. Coarse, curvilinear calcification in a pelvic mass
C. Well-defined hypoechoic mass on US
D. Well-defined mass with low signal on T2-weighted images.

Treatment

Surgical hysterectomy and multiple myomectomy are the traditional treatment offered to patients. In recent years image-guided embolisation of fibroids has emerged as another option for treatment of symptomatic uterine fibroid tumours.

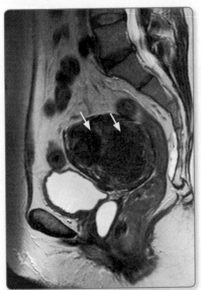

Figure 8.6 MR scan showing multiple fibroids within the uterus as hypointense rounded lesions (arrows).

8.4 Ovarian cancer

Most ovarian neoplasms are epithelial in origin and include serous, mucinous, endometrioid, undifferentiated and clear cell subtypes. They usually carry a poor prognosis and spread in the abdominopelvic cavity. It usually affects postmenopausal women and presents with vague symptoms such as swelling or pain in the abdomen, shortness of breath, unexplained weight gain, or changes in bowel or bladder habits.

Key facts

Ovarian cancers are bilateral in 20–40% of cases and present late, with disease already present outside the ovary in 75% of patients.

Radiological findings

Radiograph Large tumours may be seen on radiographs as soft-tissue masses displacing bowel loops (**Figure 8.7**). Hazy, granular calcification may be present in a subtype of ovarian tumours called serous cystadenocarcinomas.

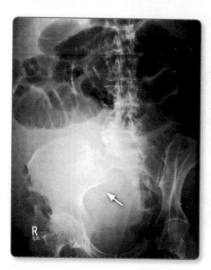

Figure 8.7 Radiograph showing a large pelvic mass displacing and obstructing small bowel loop. Note the absence of fat lines and margins, suggestive of extensive ascites (arrow).

US Ascites is common. Tumours are typically cystic with multiple septations and solid elements (**Figure 8.8**). The solid elements may show increased vascularity on Doppler scans. TVUS provides better anatomical and Doppler information compared with transabdominal US.

CT/MRI CT and MRI assist in staging of the tumour and metastases. CT shows multicystic mass with calcification, ascites and peritoneal thickening in advanced disease (**Figure 8.9**). MRI is superior in detecting local invasion of the bladder, vagina or pelvic wall (**Figure 8.10**). Omental cake (thickening due to metastases) and peritoneal seedling deposits are also best seen on CT.

Key imaging findings
A. Pelvic mass
B. Multicystic pelvic mass with solid elements and septations
C. Ascites
D. Omental and peritoneal thickening

Treatment
Surgical excision or chemotherapy.

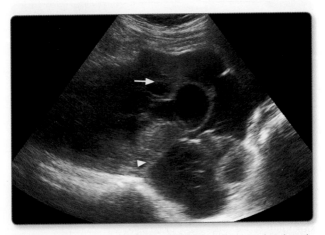

Figure 8.8 US scan showing a multicystic pelvic mass with hypoechoic (arrow) and solid echogenic areas (arrowhead).

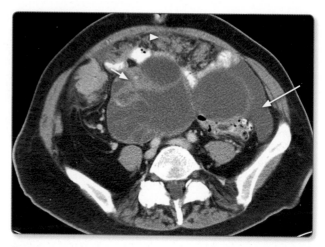

Figure 8.9 CT scan showing ovarian cancer, seen as a multicystic mass with solid enhancing areas (short arrow). Omental thickening (arrowhead) and ascites (long arrow) are present.

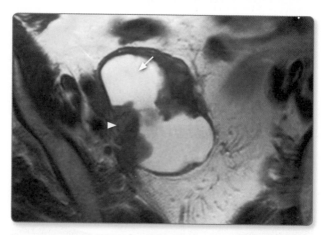

Figure 8.10 MR scan shows ovarian cancer with greater accuracy: the solid areas (arrowhead) are more easily differentiated from cystic elements (arrow).

8.5 Ovarian cysts

Ovarian non-neoplastic cysts are the most common lesions to occur in the ovary. Cysts can be functional/simple, which are associated with hormone production and occur during ovulation, or they may be non-functioning. Almost all premenopausal women have ovarian cysts whereas they occur in up to 15% of postmenopausal women. Physiological cysts can be follicular or haemorrhagic (corpus luteum) cysts.

Key facts
- Physiological ovarian cysts are commonly seen in menstruating woman but may be seen in postmenopausal women
- A mature graafian follicle is seen in the midcycle and may normally reach a size of approximately 20 mm
- After ovulation, haemorrhage causes formation of a corpus luteum cyst which may be up to 3 cm in size
- Unilocular cysts up to 3 cm may be seen in women who have no problems.

Radiological findings

US Follicular cysts have a small, thin wall and are anechoic (**Figure 8.11**). Corpus luteum cysts are caused by haemorrhage and tend to be unilocular, although they contain echogenic thrombus and fluid levels. The most important predictor of a benign cyst is a unilocular structure with thin walls. Identification of haemorrhage in a unilocular cyst is also good evidence of a benign lesion (**Figure 8.12**).

Key imaging findings
A. Unilocular cyst
B. Size <30 mm
C. Thin walls
D. Haemorrhagic content

Treatment
Symptomatic treatment.

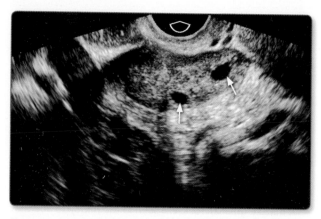

Figure 8.11 Transvaginal US showing normal ovarian cysts as unilocular hypoechoic lesions (arrows).

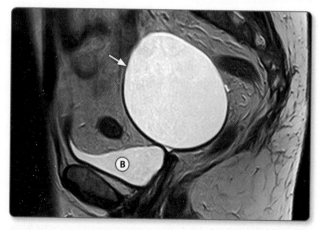

Figure 8.12 MR scan showing a large simple ovarian cyst, seen as a unilocular lesion with no septation or solid elements (arrow). **B** bladder.

8.6 Pelvic inflammatory disease

Pelvic inflammatory disease (PID) is an inflammation of the fallopian tubes and ovaries. Extragenital causes, including diverticulitis, Crohn's disease and appendicitis, may mimic PID or cause inflammation of genital organs by contiguous spread of infection.

Key facts

- Acute inflammation of the fallopian tubes is commonly due to *Chlamydia* species or gonococci
- Adhesions may form at the fimbrial end of the tube after infection, leading to tubal distension
- The distended tube may be filled with serous fluid (hydrosalpinx) or pus (pyosalpinx).

Radiological findings

Radiograph PID may cause blurring or loss of normal fat lines. Localised dilatation of the pelvic small bowel may be present.

US The uterus may appear ill defined and fluid may be present in the rectouterine pouch. Hydrosalpinx or pyosalpinx is seen as a tubular, flask-shaped structures. Pyosalpinx may show internal debris and fluid–fluid levels due to contained pus (**Figure 8.13**).

CT This may also demonstrate infected tubes with thick, enhancing walls (**Figure 8.14**).

A tubo-ovarian abscess is seen as a mass with echogenic walls and a sonolucent centre. Septations may be present within the abscess. Ureteric obstruction occurs in most patients with adnexal abscesses (80%) and this may be seen as hydronephrosis on US or CT.

Key imaging findings

A. Free fluid in rectouterine pouch
B. Tubular cystic structure in the adnexal region
C. Pyosalpinx has fluid levels and debris
D. Hydronephrosis due to ureteric obstruction in tubo-ovarian abscesses.

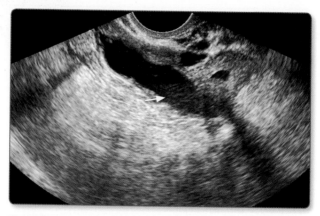

Figure 8.13 Tubo-ovarian abscess seen on transvaginal US as cystic, tubular structures containing echogenic debris (arrow).

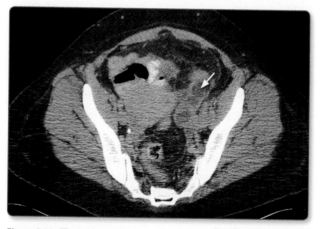

Figure 8.14 CT scan showing an enhancing, multiloculated tubular structure (arrow) in the pelvis on the left side, with surrounding inflammation. This was a pyosalpinx.

Treatment

Treatment is based on antibiotic therapy to control the infection. In advanced cases surgical excision may be required.

Miscellaneous disorders

Miscellaneous disorders of the abdomen include conditions not related to any specific organ group and include entities such as ascites, lymphadenopathy, hernias and vascular aneurysms. A variety of imaging modalities is used in the diagnosis of these conditions.

9.1 Abscess (intra-abdominal)

Intra-abdominal abscesses are localised collections of pus that are confined in the peritoneal cavity by an inflammatory barrier, including the omentum, inflammatory adhesions or contiguous viscera.

Patients may present with abdominal pain, focal tenderness, spiking fever, prolonged ileus and leukocytosis.

Key facts

Abdominal abscesses have many causes, the common ones being bowel perforation, appendicitis, diverticulitis, pancreatitis and spread of abdominal wall infections.

Radiological findings

Radiograph Findings may include a localised ileus, extraluminal gas and air–fluid levels (**Figure 9.1**). Pleural effusions may be present in subphrenic (under diaphragm) collections.

US Appearances vary from being cyst like to even solid masses. Most have a hypoechoic centre (due to purulent fluid) and contain fluid levels. Debris within the abscess may have strong echoes. Gas-containing abscesses may be echogenic, and abscesses are generally ovoid and have an irregular wall.

CT CT has >95% accuracy in the detection of abscesses. The appearance of an air bubble or fluid levels within a fluid collection or a low-attenuation extraluminal mass is diagnostic of an intra-abdominal collection. Abscesses typically show ring enhancement of their margins (**Figure 9.2**).

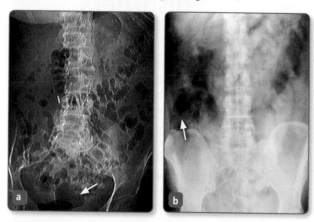

Figure 9.1 Intra-abdominal abscesses can be seen as abnormal gas collections or fluid levels. Radiographs showing (a) extraluminal gas seen adjacent to be sigmoid and rectum (arrow), and (b) mottled gas lucencies not conforming to any bowel segment seen in the right lumbar quadrant (arrow).

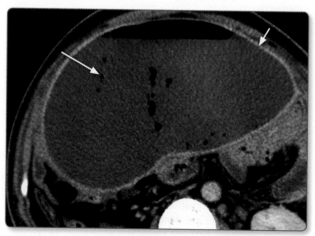

Figure 9.2 CT scan of a large abscess containing gas and fluid levels (long arrow). Note the typical rim enhancement of the abscess margins (short arrow).

Key imaging findings

A. Extraluminal gas
B. Hypoechoic mass with debris or gas
C. Fluid levels or gas within a collection
D. Enhancing margins

Treatment

Antibiotic treatment or drainage of the abscess.

9.2 Abdominal aneurysm

Most abdominal aortic aneurysms (AAAs) are acquired and secondary to atherosclerosis. Over 95% of AAAs are distal to the origin of the renal arteries. Patients may be asymptomatic or a pulsatile mass may be palpated in the upper abdomen. The prevalence of AAAs increases with age, with an average age of 65–70 at the time of diagnosis.

Key facts

- Elastin, the principal load-bearing protein present in the wall of the aorta, is less abundant in the abdominal aorta compared with the thoracic aorta
- The abdominal aorta does not possess vasa vasorum, hindering repair
- Aneurysms <5 cm have low risk of rupture
- Larger AAAs >6 cm have a natural tendency to expand and up to a quarter of these aneurysms may rupture within 5 years.

Radiological findings

Radiograph A soft-tissue shadow obscuring the renal and psoas shadows, particularly on the left side, may be seen on radiographs. Curvilinear calcification in the aneurysmal wall is often present (**Figure 9.3**).

US/CT The criterion for diagnosis of an AAA is a diameter >3 cm on US or CT. Aneurysms appear as saccular or fusiform dilatation of the aorta. Calcification may be seen along the aortic wall. Often the aneurysm contains thrombus, which is of low echogenicity on US and does not show enhancement on CT (**Figure 9.4**).

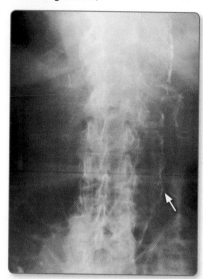

Figure 9.3 Radiograph showing the calcified wall of an abdominal aortic aneurysm as a curvilinear area of density along the spine (arrow).

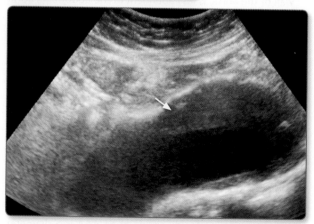

Figure 9.4 US scan showing abdominal aortic aneurysm with contained echogenic thrombus (arrow)

Key imaging findings

A. Soft-tissue shadow obscuring renal and psoas margins
B. Curvilinear calcification
C. Fusiform or saccular shape
D. Contained thrombus

Treatment

Larger aneurysms may require endovascular stenting or surgical repair.

9.3 Ascites

Fluid can accumulate in the peritoneal cavity (ascites – Greek: askos = bag/sac) for a variety of reasons, including cirrhosis (75%), malignancy (15%), heart failure (3%), tuberculosis (TB – 2%) and pancreatitis (1%). On examination, it can be detected above approximately 1500 ml, presenting with bulging of the flanks in the supine position and 'shifting dullness' to percussion.

Key facts

• Ascites can be transudative or exudative in nature
• Transudates are a result of increased pressure in the portal vein (>8 mm Hg) and the fluid is essentially 'ultrafiltrated plasma' through normal capillaries
• Exudates are actively secreted fluid due to inflammation or malignancy.

Radiological findings

US Fluid (as little as 10–15 ml) can be detected at the inferior edge of the liver in the supine position (hepatorenal pouch) and the pelvic cul de sac. Typical serous ascites appears as hypoechoic fluid surrounding abdominal organs (**Figures 9.5 and 9.6**). Small bowel loops will appear suspended within the ascitic fluid, tethered to the mesenteric leaves, and form a 'fan appearance'. Debris may be seen in exudative fluid due to proteinaceous content.

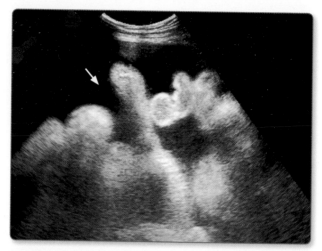

Figure 9.5 US scan showing ascites as hypoechoic fluid collection in the abdomen. The mesentery and bowel loops appear to be floating within the fluid (arrow).

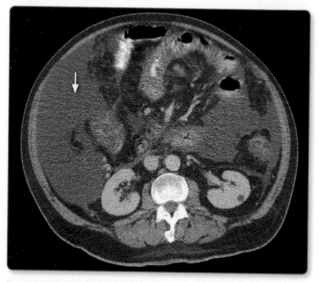

Figure 9.6 CT scan of ascites showing a fluid collection (arrow) in the sub-hepatic region surrounding the bowel loops.

Key imaging findings

A. Free fluid in the hepatorenal pouch
B. Fan appearance
C. Triangular cap of fluid over the uterus
D. Debris in exudative ascites

Treatment

Drainage of ascites.

9.4 Abdominal hernias

An external abdominal hernia occurs when the contents of the peritoneal cavity (e.g. intestines or mesenteric fat) bulge out at areas of abdominal wall weakness. They need to be diagnosed early because they can cause strangulation or closed loop obstruction that needs emergency surgery. Presentation of symptomatic hernias may range from minor discomfort to clinically serious bowel obstruction with strangulation.

Key facts

Most hernias are in the groin and can be inguinal (75% of all hernias) or femoral.

Radiological findings

Radiograph Hernias may occasionally be seen (**Figure 9.7**).

US This can also be used for detecting abdominal hernias. The main advantage is that scanning can be done while the patient increases abdominal pressure to highlight the (transient) hernia, by coughing or Valsalva's manoeuvre.

CT This is useful in the delineation of hernias. Inguinal hernias can be indirect or direct. Indirect hernias are more common (two thirds of all abdominal hernias), and occur through a patent processus vaginalis, so that the hernial sac is lateral to the inferior epigastric vessels. Direct inguinal hernias are caused by acquired weakness of the transversalis fascia (the membrane between the transverse abdominal muscle and extraperitoneal fascia), so the hernial sac is located medial to the inferior epigastric vessels (**Figure 9.8**). Femoral hernias are more common

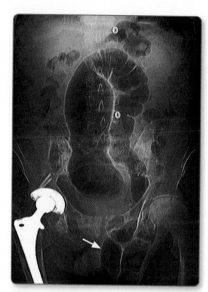

Figure 9.7 Radiograph showing an inguinal hernia containing gas filled large bowel loop (arrow).

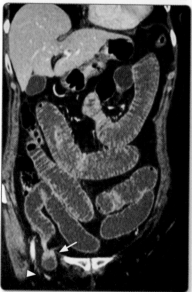

Figure 9.8 CT scan showing an inguinal hernia containing small bowel (arrow). This hernia is medial to the inferior epigastric vessels (arrowhead) and is therefore a direct hernia. CT shows the narrow neck of the hernia to good advantage, which predicts possible complications such as strangulation.

in women and arise from a defect in the attachment of the transversalis fascia to the pubis and so are posterior to the inguinal ligament and medial to the femoral vessels. Parastomal hernias (e.g. after a colostomy) may contain a large length of bowel and present with intermittent obstructive features.

Key imaging findings

A. Indirect inguinal hernia lateral to epigastric vessels
B. Direct inguinal hernia medial to epigastric vessels
C. Femoral hernia medial to femoral vessels
D. Parastomal hernia present adjacent to the stoma

Treatment

Surgical correction.

9.5 Lymphoma

Lymphomas form up to 5% of all adult malignancies, and usually present with widespread lymphadenopathy. Extranodal involvement is usually seen in those with widespread nodal disease, although it can also be the initial sign. Patients may present with lymphadenopathy, generalised malaise, fever, night sweats or vague symptoms.

Key facts

- Lymphoma is classified into two broad groups: Hodgkin's disease and non-Hodgkin's lymphoma (NHL)
- Hodgkin's disease commonly involves the nodes of the neck and shoulders (80–90%)
- The lymph nodes of the chest are often affected, and these may be noticed on a chest radiograph
- NHL is up to eight times more common than Hodgkin's disease and the most common subtype is diffuse large B-cell lymphoma (DLBCL), an aggressive, high-grade disease
- Extranodal disease is common in NHL, and usually seen in the liver, kidney, lung or bone marrow
- The second most common type of NHL is follicular lymphoma, which is less aggressive.

Radiological findings

CT This is used to provide staging and follow-up of lymphoma. Enlarged abdominal nodes (>15 mm) can be seen as rounded, nodular structures in the mesentery and retroperitoneum. Often there is hepatosplenomegaly. Focal lesions of the liver and spleen may be present, which are typically hypodense. The spleen is more commonly involved and usually splenic lesions are associated with lymphadenopathy at the splenic hilum.

Extensive mesenteric lymphadenopathy forms the 'sandwich sign' of low-density nodes surrounding high-density mesenteric vessels (**Figure 9.9**).

The gastrointestinal (GI) tract is the most common extranodal site of involvement of NHL, particularly the small bowel. Small bowel lymphoma causes marked bowel wall thickening. Aneurysmal dilatation of the bowel may be present due to destruction of the muscle layers by lymphomatous involvement.

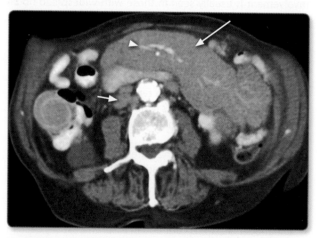

Figure 9.9 CT scan showing extensive lymphadenopathy in the mesentery (long arrow) as a confluent mass. The encased mesenteric blood vessels (arrowhead) appear as linear densities forming the sandwich sign. Para-aortic lymph nodes are also present (short arrow).

Key imaging findings
A. Enlarged lymph nodes
B. Sandwich sign
C. Marked circumferential thickening of the bowel in GI lymphoma
D. Hepatosplenomegaly with/without focal lesions

Treatment

Treatment is based on symptomatic radiotherapy and chemotherapy for low-grade NHL and aggressive chemotherapy for high-grade NHL. Localised Hodgkin's disease is usually managed with radiotherapy, whereas advanced disease requires chemotherapy as well.

9.6 Penetrating and projectile injuries

Blunt and penetrating abdominal trauma such as that resulting from road traffic accidents or projectile (bullet, shrapnel) and sharp weapons (knives) can cause significant injury to the solid organs, blood vessels and bowel. Presentation may be with hypovolaemic shock (due to blood loss) and peritonitis. Stab wounds to the anterior abdomen are associated with a 30–50% and gunshot injuries with a 90% incidence of intra-abdominal organ injury which requires surgical repair.

Key facts

- Projectile injuries are categorised by the location of the entrance and exit wounds
- Penetrating injuries enter the body but do not exit
- Penetrating trauma can be life threatening because abdominal organs can bleed profusely
- Large organs such as the liver have significant blood supply, so injuries lead to greater blood loss.

Radiological findings

CT This provides the most accurate evidence of intra-abdominal injuries in perforating and projectile injuries. Wound tracks through soft tissue are characterised by fluid, blood or gas collections, and pneumoperitoneum is particularly evident in cases with bowel injury (**Figure 9.10**). Traffic injuries can cause trauma to solid organs, leading to contusions and lacerations, which appear as branching or linear areas of non-enhancement on CT. Seat-belt and traffic injuries can also cause superficial injuries to the subcutaneous tissues (**Figure 9.11**). In cases with projectile injury, foreign materials within the body (e.g. bullets, metallic fragments or other material) are noted on radiographs or CT scans (**Figure 9.12**). Foreign bodies such as bullets or shrapnel are usually hyperdense on CT. CT has high accuracy in detecting peritoneum breach, which is seen as fluid collections and haemoperitoneum (hyperdense fluid).

Key imaging findings

A. Foreign body in the abdomen

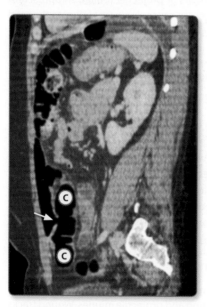

Figure 9.10 CT scan in a patient with a stab wound. There is perforation of the colon ⓒ with an anterior collection of air (arrow).

B. Pneumoperitoneum
C. Haemoperitoneum
D. Solid organ laceration or contusions

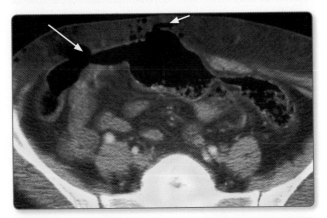

Figure 9.11 CT scan showing disruption of the anterior abdominal muscles (long arrow) and perforation of the colon (short arrow).

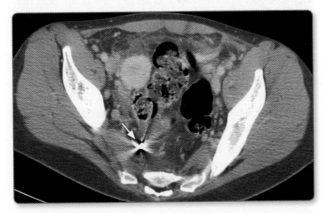

Figure 9.12 CT scan showing a bullet as a hyperdense lesion (arrow). A projectile track is seen behind the bullet.

9.7 Adrenal tumours – phaeochromocytomas

Phaeochromocytomas arise from chromaffin cells of the adrenal medulla and secrete excessive amounts of catecholamines, usually adrenaline. The incidence is estimated at 2–8 cases per 1000,000 population. Presentation may be with a hypertensive crisis associated with pain, tremors, fever and sweating.

Key facts

- Ninety per cent arise from the adrenal glands whereas the rest are extra-adrenal
- Ten per cent are bilateral and 10% are associated with syndromes such as von Hippel–Lindau syndrome, multiple endocrine neoplasia (MEN) type II, tuberous sclerosis or neurofibromatosis.

Radiological findings

CT or MRI is used for detection and staging of phaeochromocytomas.

CT Heterogeneous density and up to 7–8% of tumours may demonstrate calcification. Tumours show intense contrast enhancement due to hypervascularity, often with central areas of low density representing tumour necrosis.

MRI Very bright on T2-weighted sequences (**Figure 9.13**); areas of high signal may also be seen on T1-weighted images due to haemorrhage. On post-contrast images a 'salt-and-pepper' appearance is seen due to the presence of enhancing tumour (bright) interspersed with multiple tiny blood vessels (dark).

Nuclear imaging Using ^{123}I-labelled meta-iodobenzylguanidine (MIBG) scan nuclear imaging can be used to detect tumour uptake and also uptake in metastases or recurrent tumours.

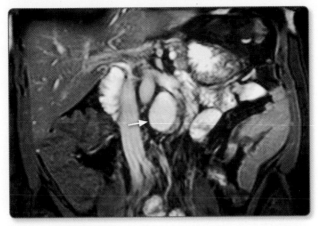

Figure 9.13 Hyperintense lesion (arrow) seen involving the left adrenal due to phaeochromocytoma.

Key imaging findings
A. Heterogeneous, hypervascular tumours on CT
B. Bright signal on T2-weighted MRI
C. 'Salt-and-pepper' appearance
D. Uptake on MIBG scans

Treatment
Surgical resection.

Bibliography

Adam A, Dixon AK, Grainger RG, Allison DJ, Eds. Grainger & Allison's Diagnostic Radiology, 5th edn. Edinburgh: Churchill Livingstone; 2007.

Allan PL, Baxter GM, Weston MJ. Clinical Ultrasound, 3rd edn. London, Churchill Livingstone; 2011.

Balthazar EJ, Herlinger H, Maglinte D, Birnbaum BA. Clinical Imaging of the Small Intestine, 2nd edn. New York: Springer; 2001.

Gore RM, Levine MS. Textbook of Gastrointestinal Radiology, 3rd edn. Philadelphia: Saunders; 2007.

Russell RCG, Williams NS, Bulstrode CJK. Bailey and Love's Short Practice of Surgery, 25th edn. London: Hodder Arnold; 2008.

Sinnatamby CS. Last's Anatomy: Regional and Applied, 10th edn. Edinburgh: Churchill Livingstone; 1999.

Stevenson GW, Freeny PC, Margulis AR, Burhenne HJ. Margulis and Burhenne's Alimentary Tract Radiology, 5th edn. St Louis: Mosby-Year Book; 1994.

Index

Note: Page references followed by the letter f indicate illustrations, e.g. 214f.